Dedicated to all the
women and chilc  he

"It genuinely has made me laugh and cry in equal measures... Thank you for so skilfully articulating my story and giving me a voice."

<small>SWAN WHO WAS LOVELIER THAN HE TOLD HER</small>

"There's some of it that is still very hard to read in the same way it was hard to live. But as well as the tough bits, there were bits that made me smile and bits that made me laugh out loud."

<small>JILL WHO ESCAPED THE BEANSTALK</small>

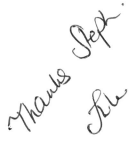

Cataloguing-in-Publication Data
A catalogue record for this book is available
from the British Library
ISBN 978-1-9996624-0-0

Published by Middle Farm Press
Author: Julie Leoni © 2018
Illustrator: Anita Wyatt © 2018
Managing Editor: Kate Taylor
Designer: Su Richards
Printed in the UK by Think Digital Books Ltd
Legal review by Alex Wade of Cleared and Reviewed
Cover photograph © Sebastian Parfitt, illustrated by Anita Wyatt ©

MIDDLE
FARM
PRESS

Contents

Forewords

THIS IS AN ENCHANTING BOOK of fairy tales, full of wisdom and courage and fear and doubt. The tales weave together darkness, violence, captivity and torture with goodness, light, escape and healing.

These are tales, told by real women about the domestic abuse they have suffered. Julie Leoni's unique story-telling approach to these real-life accounts has the combined effect of heightening the horror of what happened to the women, whilst at the same time allowing the illusion of the 'fairy tale' to provide some emotional distance and safety.

Being a victim of domestic abuse can leave you with enduring low self-esteem, self-doubt, an inability to trust yourself and others, emotional detachment and anxiety. Telling your story is not easy. I know, because I too have my own story.

As an experienced coach and facilitator of hundreds of women's development programmes, I know the healing power of being with people who are willing to share their experiences with you and to be with you without judgement.

I honour the author and all the women in this book who had the courage to tell their stories so that others in the same situation can know that they are not alone and that there is hope and wisdom from those who have walked into, and out of the woods before them.

I hope this book is read, shared, talked of, written about and passed from woman to woman. I hope it inspires more women to tell their stories and to grow in courage and strength. I hope it inspires women to support one other, to ask for help, to value themselves, to learn to put themselves first and to turn darkness into light.

I hope it saves some lives.

KIM MORGAN MCC, MA., DIRECTOR BAREFOOT COACHING LTD, AUTHOR THE COACH'S CASEBOOK, COACH, COACH TRAINER, KEYNOTE SPEAKER.
HTTPS://WWW.BAREFOOTCOACHING.CO.UK

WHEN I WAS maybe 4 or 5 years old a kind Aunt gifted me a huge hardbacked book of Grimm's Fairy tales. I recall many a rainy day flicking through the colourful illustrated pages, entertaining myself retelling the stories in my own words.

Retelling classic stories isn't something new however, it takes a highly talented author to take real life examples of modern day abuse, co-dependence and domestic violence and rewrite them as classic fairy tales.

Into the Woods ingeniously combines self-help with magic and fantasy. This nurturing collection of tales shines light on these dark, seldom spoken about experiences to create a healing, informing and empowering resource.

I defy any woman not to relate to at least one of the characters in these carefully crafted tales, uniting women in their woe, to reclaim their power and potential.

May these tales provide courage, hope and an opportunity for change and in doing so awaken future generations of women to their full potential.

An absolute must read for women everywhere.

ALLISON MARLOWE FOUNDER OF GLOBAL WINNING WOMEN, COACH, PIONEER OF THE NEW FEMININE PARADIGM, ALLISONMARLOWE.COM

THESE STORIES are spell-binding: harsh legacies and histories, painful recovery and hopeful futures. Through the genre of the fairy story, Into the Woods succeeds in helping us to understand something very important about the vulnerability and cruelty of human nature.

Based on life histories, these are a very cleverly drawn set of stories that leave us both horrified and compassionate. The women are not without flaws nor are the men, the perpetrators, intrinsically evil yet we are taken through the human suffering and despair of the kind that far too many women experience.

Into the Woods shows women how to find their power, first individually and then, collectively through fierce love, deep courage, tentative hope and commitment to the hard work of recovery and healing.

Storytelling and therapy combined.

DR ANNE-MARIE WRIGHT EdD, MA (SEN), BED HONS, PGDIP PSYCHOANALYTIC OBSERVATIONAL STUDIES, LECTURER AND CONSULTANT WORKING WITH VULNERABLE CHILDREN AND ADULTS WITH TRAUMA.

Introduction

THIS IS A BOOK about domestic abuse. It is the book I looked for and couldn't find when I was leaving an abusive relationship. This is the book I needed to help me understand why I, a woman with a PhD, a career in education, emotional intelligence and a large circle of friends, had ended up in the relationship I did. This is the book I needed to help me forgive myself and to heal. This is the book I needed so I knew I wasn't alone, that there wasn't something fatally flawed in me, that I wasn't doomed. This is the book I needed to give me hope.

This book has taken some time to write. Leaving a relationship, any relationship, is hard. So much harder when your confidence is on the floor and you are scared about the consequences of your leaving. I could not have written it sooner.

The only thing I wrote during the early months after leaving, was my own story, for myself, that no one else would read. I wrote it as a dark fairy tale, full of foreshadowed threat and danger. It was the only way I could write about my experience. To describe it in black and white on a page in any other way was too frightening, too raw.

I needed the fairy tale structure to give my experience form, to give it shape. I needed to make him, my ex, simpler, more one-dimensional and a little less real. To write about him in a realistic way was daunting, so I chose this way to make sense and meaning of the darkness and to give shape to the chaos that had swirled around me during those years. Writing my story gave me some comfort; gave me back some of my lost control. I was in charge of the narrative in stark contrast to the way I had felt controlled in the relationship.

Once I had steadied myself into my new life, I attended the Freedom Programme and got one-to-one support to understand and debrief not only what had happened to me personally, but to put it in a framework to understand how abuse works. I found a therapist who taught me, reminded me, ordered me, to put my own needs at a level with everyone else's, to elevate them from under the table to at least taking a seat at the table of needs being met. She helped me forgive myself for not spotting what I couldn't have recognised because I had never seen it before; I had no map, no compass, and I was so tuned out from my own intuition that I hadn't noticed how wrong the relationship had felt.

The more I understood, the lighter I felt. I felt safer and reassured that I wouldn't repeat the pattern again. It was critical for me to understand how I had fallen for him, why I hadn't spotted the signs, why it took me so long to leave. Getting the support allowed me to let go of some of the enormous burden of shame I felt. Shame and self-recrimination at what I had allowed myself to tolerate, and shame that I hadn't known better.

I know that domestic abuse is also experienced by men and I acknowledge and respect their experience as I do the experience of women. However, I am not a man, nor have I heard the tales of men who have been abused. Women's tales are the only ones I feel qualified to tell.

Hearing other women's stories in the groups I attended was humbling; many had suffered horrendous physical and sexual abuse as well as the emotional and psychological abuse which is always present. As I sat in those circles and saw the dark-ringed, downturned eyes, the grey skin, the shaking hands, the stooped shoulders, I felt awe at what these women did to keep their kids safe, to keep themselves safe and to make it through each day.

I also felt anger. Why had no one taught us about this stuff? Why isn't The Freedom Programme taught in schools to help us avoid abusive relationships in the first place, rather than to help people escape from them much later? My anger was also at the legal traps I heard about; the solicitors who didn't know enough about abuse and so didn't place the court orders when they should have. My anger was at a legal system that seemed to favour the rights of the fathers, no matter what they had done, over the rights of the children and mothers trying to keep their children safe.

In the years since, as a coach, I have worked with women and girls who are in abusive relationships because they didn't spot the signs before they were in too deep. I have heard stories of schools that did nothing when pupils told them how daddy hits mummy. I have heard stories about women who couldn't leave because they had no money and no job and nowhere to go. There is such a lack of public awareness as to how abuse works. It is this need to educate as well as my need to make sense of what happened to me which has led me to write this book.

I wanted to hear other women's stories from start to finish, rather than just the fragments I picked up at work or in the groups, which is why I interviewed the women in these stories. I am a qualitative researcher, and interviews are my home ground for understanding real, messy, lived experiences. I emailed the questions I wanted to ask along with the consent forms, and sent both the transcripts and the actual interviews back to the women to review. When I had completed the first full draft I sent it to all the women and waited; excited at what I hoped would be an empowering and enlightening read for them all.

One woman felt empowered to have her story heard and believed, another woman edited what she had said to clarify and expand on it, but the other responses surprised me. One of the women withdrew entirely and other women couldn't bring themselves to reread their own stories. I spoke to one of the women in more detail who explained: she had never told the story all in one go before and she felt like the telling of it had been a relief and offered healing. She had felt better for having told me her story. However, when I asked her to read my first draft, she couldn't face it: she panicked and felt sick, literally and then metaphorically. Telling her story had been like vomiting all the bad stuff out of her system; and then to be asked to reread it was like being asked to eat her own bile: it felt too horrific to consider. This explained a lot. Why would you want to reread your own words about a time in your life which was so painful?

So I changed how it was written; I turned away from the more academic tone of the first draft to the fairy tale form which had helped me. I wanted to write an easily accessible book so that anyone can learn about domestic abuse and how to spot it, avoid it or get out of it. If you are living with domestic abuse now, I want you to know that you are not alone, you are not all the things you are being told you are, and there is hope; I want to you to hear other people's stories. I believe it will help.

Fairy tales were part of my childhood; princes, princesses, white horses and high turrets. The prince was always handsome, brave, honest and devoted, willing to cut through thorns and climb up towers to reach his true love. The princess was young, virginal, obedient; either loved by all or the victim of some parental evil. She would remain pure of mind and deed no matter what trials she suffered, endlessly forgiving, patient and kind. She would wait, passively, for life to unroll around her; she need take no action, learn no skills, for at some point, she would be saved by a man. I loved them. I wanted to be carried off by Donny Osmond on a charger. I wanted a fairy godmother to help with my O' levels and to somehow mend my parents' failing marriage. I wanted to be found by my own true love.

I have sons, and it slowly dawned on me as I read to them night after night, that fairy tales are aimed at girls; there are no fairy stories for boys. My boys hated all that princess-waiting-with-flowers-and-slumber stuff. Instead we read action adventure stories, naughty boy stories, boys and dinosaurs stories. In these stories, the boys are active, curious, adventurous, brave, courageous, rebellious, sharp, perceptive, quick-witted, strong and agile. They aced it every time; all wounds healed, all beasts slain, all girls (if there were any) lead masterfully into their second place.

Sigh.

Women have tales to tell, voices to be heard, victories to be celebrated, courage to be recognised, healing to be done, meaning to be carved. I came across Viktor Frankl when I was doing my coaching training. He wrote Man's Search for Meaning after surviving the Nazi concentration camps. In it he says that we all have a fundamental need to make meaning of what happens to us: '*Striving to find meaning in one's life is the primary motivational source in man*' and that when we make that meaning, it is ours, we claim it and no one can take it away from us unless we let them.

'*Everything can be taken from a man but one thing; the last of human freedoms – to choose one's attitude in any given set of circumstances... If there is to be meaning in life at all, then there must be a meaning in suffering*'. Frankl, V. E. (2004) Man's Search For Meaning, Rider, London, pages 75,76 and 104

When we tell our story, we shape, narrate, describe and make sense of it and this gives us back some of the power we lost. Telling our story is healing. I believe that all humans have the desire to pass our stories on, to feel that somehow our stories might help other people, that somehow, we might be heard and seen and that our stories might live on beyond our flesh and bones. Sharing our stories allows us to change something bad into something good, to reclaim our voice, to put order and structure where there was none, to take the base metal of lived experience and to transform it into gold. Stories can heal and free the tellers as well as those to whom the stories are told.

All the women in this book had stories which they could not tell at the time. Their stories need passing on so that there is a greater understanding amongst the police, the legal system, schools, neighbours and loved ones, who simply can't understand why people living with abuse 'don't just leave'.

We need new womanish stories for ourselves, our mothers and fathers, our grandparents, our daughters and sons, nieces and nephews, grandchildren, pupils and friends. We need new fairy stories, witches' stories, wise woman stories, tales of female bravery and valour found in chipped cups and the laundry basket as well as in the dark, tangled forest paths of our inner world and relationships.

The witches of old were ordinary women who were accused and convicted of and killed for acts they could not prove themselves innocent of. They were often women who spoke back to power; disturbing the status quo, challenging male authority. We see the same in the #Me Too movement today where some commentators see women as the problem and label them slags and whores, accusing them of instigating witch hunts against the male perpetrators.

The women in these stories were called names they did not deserve and harmed in often unimaginable ways for unnamed 'crimes' they didn't understand and were innocent of. Let us now reclaim that name-calling and re-empower ourselves. Let us take back 'witch' for our own, for there is a power in women that we don't always allow ourselves to know.

The women who told the tales you are about to read have battled danger and protected the weak, they have defended Hope and clung on to Sanity. They have walked in the dark of the new moon, faced the wolves' jaws, found their way into the depth of the forest, into the fire, and are ready to speak their truth.

Hear their howls.

Make your way into the midnight womb of the forest, look to the moon for direction and you will find us in circles around our flames. There is nothing to fear for we will guide you in and guide you safely out of the clearing of your lives, but not before we have passed on the treasure of our wisdom; that you may be wiser, more alert, more discerning, more able to trust your gut and wield your own sword to fend off dragons. More able to be your own hero.

Gather close to hear these witches' tales.

The fire is burning.

Come and join us.

Sleeping Beauty

ONCE UPON A TIME there lived a very happy family, in a very happy house, in a nothing-special town, in a recovering-from-war land. The mother had escaped the bomb-scarred gas of Europe, leaving nightmares of her Jewish ghosts in ghettos, camps and ovens. Shushed and hushed and hidden as a child she had learned to keep her head down and her mouth shut, to pass invisibly through the crowds of baying hounds hunting her tribe down from Florence to Naples, from Anzio to Rome. If cornered she would roll over, submissive, cowed – cowering but not cowardly. She had lost so much, so many; fingers could neither count nor minds contain the multitude of shoes and combs and pans piled high in silent, impersonal memorial to the nameless millions.

No wonder then, that the life she built in this bland, English town was small and safe and quiet. Silently, sliding through life, grateful for not causing noses to sniff or heads to turn.

Until she met him, and his head did turn.

His head did turn, his heart did pound, his hands did sweat and his breathing quicken. It was the clichéd love at first sight, with all the divided tension of Romeo and Juliet – for he was not a Yid, nor a spic, nor a wop, nor a dago, just a terribly decent English chap.

Tricky.

She hid her Jewishness from the world as best she could, but not from him and when their religions and their faiths tried to pull them asunder, they flung the Bible and the Torah to the winds and reached for love, for each other. A mixed-race marriage dare not darken the doors of church or synagogue so it was in a dusty, fusty civic office where they plighted their troths and escaped quickly home to the warmth and passion of their bed.

But people talked, as they do, suspicious in the rebuilding of their own ruins. Often he or she would face the scowling gesticulations of blitz babies, or duck the missiled eggs or stones of those who trusted no one, whose love was strictly rationed to their own; tolerance blacked out. They would scuttle homeward, heads bowed in obeisance and sorrow to fall into each other's outstretched limbs.

So no wonder that when her belly swelled they used all their might to block out the cruelty and suffering of their worlds, to keep their youngsters safe and cushioned from the bashes and bruises to create a quiet life. A boy was born, and then a girl, welcomed with delight and awe that such fragile beauty should spring from such haunted loins. They were stroked and rocked, lullabied and washed, kissed and inhaled, caressed and attended to with such alertness that the babes wanted for nothing, had to ask for nothing, were scared of nothing. A sweet dream of a childhood.

The mother cooked as Jewish Italian mothers do; with love in every mouthful, with passion in every portion, imbued with the scents of succulence and the tastes of tenderness. The father worked hard and when the mother wanted to grow and earn, he supported her graduation and career, never telling her that she belonged at home shackled to sink or sofa. He was a liberal, a feminist, long before such words were used, weird and ahead of his time. When all the other mothers had on their pinnies and were baking apple pies whilst quaffing down mother's little helpers, this mother was studying and working and raising children in her warm embrace.

They didn't fit in; strangers, foreigners, doing it differently. The father and mother would have done anything for anyone; they liked to please, they didn't like to rock the boat or make a fuss, they kept very quiet. They painted such an idyll for their children that they lived in a rainbow world of sparkling milk and honey. Life was sweet, so sweet, like a slumbered-drowsy-dream. Sugar and spice and all things nice.

The boy and girl grew equally, what was sauce for the goose was sauce for the gander; if the boy studied, so did the girl, if the boy could work, so could the girl, if the boy could earn, so could the girl. Equal opportunities personified, embodied, inhabited and owned. The new world, the next generation, hope for us all. Happy ever after.

Until they stepped out into the mean streets, the school gates, the park benches, the back alleys; life was different there and their mother couldn't reach them, she couldn't find them or protect them and they had no shields of their own. Newly emerged from their childhood cocoon, still soft and pliant, they had no compass for the shadows, no map for the murky depths, no weapons to guard their boundaries; innocents abroad, with heads full of dreams and I heart yous; True Love.

As the son headed into his life, we follow instead the daughter; a beauty with raven hair and almond eyes, all glowing skin and open arms, kindly, cheeky and fun. She fairly bounced her way through school, Tigger-like in her enthusiasm for learning, arms linking in whispers with her friends; always up to something with their japing-jesting larks. Her head buried in books; wuthered with romance, Mockingbirded with justice, following Prospero into his isle of dreams. She wasn't looking where she was going when she bumped slap bang into him, and dropped her books, leaves scattering to the Clarked shoes of break-time-snack-rush.

She looked up and their eyes met across the crowded corridor. He scowled and wiped off the affront of her colliding, watching with a slight curl of his lip as she scrambled to collect herself and her tomes, never bending to help, presiding lord-of-the-flies-like over the blushing serf prostrated at his feet. Heart pounding, lips flushing, pupils dilating, fingers all-a-quiver, she collected herself and smiled her apologies, babbling, bumbling, blushing, bashful flirting from beneath innocently curled lashes. Her Heathcliff, her Romeo, her Odysseus at last!

As he deigned to trudge and slummock the corridor aside her impish-trip-clop dance, she inhaled his brooding-slouching-muttered monosyllables, his slightly dirty collar, his rakish-mildewed tie, the scuffs lining his slip-on shoes. He was so exotic, so other, so aloof and distant and detached.

So she fell in love, just like in the teenage mag; 'How to meet boys at the laundrette/in the library/in school'.

Her parents wanted to know every inch of her whereabouts; his didn't care. Her parents stroked and caressed, and tucked, and hugged; his grunted and shrugged from afar. She had to be in for nine, he could stay out all night. He could swear with such conviction, with words she didn't honestly understand, and she was scolded for the mildest blasphemy. She would eat with knife and forked arms, elbows off the table and tucked in; he would shove chips into his succulent, slightly drooling mouth with fag-yellowed fingers. She was Ariel to his Caliban and knew that she could train the beast, could civilise and save him; she, post-feminist-daughter would ride in on her white-emancipated-mare and save him from himself before galloping off into the golden horizon of Happy-Ever-After. Such a dream come true.

She worked hard at school, did well, pleased teachers, pleased parents, pleased her many and varied friends and pleased him. Head Girl material, the staff could never work out her attraction to Heathcliff, one of their more troublesome students; detentions here, insolence there, caught smoking yet again, not even clever enough to stub it out. A bully, he was the kind of boy who would graffiti his desk; 'Heath woz ere' and then wonder how they worked out it was him. Still, as long as she got her grades, which she did, no one interfered and her parents were much too polite and nice to share their fears.

FAST FORWARD through the first date (awkward), the first kiss (slimy), the first time he met her parents (embarrassing), the first time she met his parents (in passing), the first time they had sex (urgh, not at all like all the magazines, he clearly hadn't read Cosmo, still, maybe it would get better over time), the first day at work (she: suited-booted-polished and smart, he: in overalls, dusty, smelly), the first house they bought (or actually, that she bought, but don't mention that), her first pregnancy (working until the last minute, she was so excited. He went to the pub a lot).

But we're moving too fast. Here let's rewind a moment and take a closer look at how Beauty and her Heathcliff are faring; because, of course, she married him and so was sure to be living happily ever after.

Let's zoom in on the wedding day photograph of Heathcliff carrying his gauzy, not-quite-virgin bride across their double-glazed, newly-wed threshold. The image doesn't reveal, for the camera couldn't see, and nor could she, the sheen of dew which sprinkled, like a silken spray across her garlanded curls. So fine, it was, like a kitten's breathe whispering across her skin, tickling down her ears, inhaling and settling into her throat. The photos don't show how softly it sifted into her spirit, stilling her voice and tying her tongue. She didn't notice how quiet she had become.

His voice took up all the space.

So when he said that they should spend less, grow more, make more, she duly turned to the needles and hooks of her blanket-making grandmothers, the patchworking of hope covering the marital bed. The weeds won the battle of the aspirational vegetable patch. How could they not when she could only fight their spread on her return from work when they had all day to extend and grow. The sulky bread she made didn't want to rise and the cakes rebelled, sticking to the tins and refusing to come out. She was, as he pointed out, failing in every aspect of women's work. Of course he wouldn't sully his hands in such meniality, even though she worked longer hours and at a further stretch from him. She never thought to argue, that's not what good wives do and Beauty so wanted to be a good wife, a quiet wife.

So she didn't argue when the bills started to come in revealing his swing from slug-chewed lettuce and her stodgy macaroni cheese to only the best pre-packed food that her money could buy. She worried, but didn't say, that they couldn't afford to keep eating out or getting takeaways. She swallowed her voice with every mouthful of monosodium glutamate and practiced tolerance and acceptance as all good girls should, as he ploughed, drooling-mouthed through daytime TV, into the soaps and through the night, grunting only to point to the kitchen where she would scuttle and prepare some snack which could be eaten without having to remove his hand from the remote or his eyes from the screen.

So she was pleased when he first announced that he would swim the channel to show her and the world his Neptunian talents. This, from a man she'd never seen swim at all. He abandoned his chair and polystyrene food for the leisure centre where he swore he swam first tens, then hundreds and soon thousands of lengths a day. She enjoyed the quiet of the house his absence left, the simple routine she could establish without his endless demands.

But not for long. Soon he required high-energy food, high carbs, lean protein, an ever-changing training diet to help his newly toned (he told her) physique. Soon she became an expert in nutrition, sports massage, and motivating the sporting best (he told her) and all with her work clothes still on, quietly doing it all, having it all, living the eighties-feminist dream.

She never knew the truth of his beaching but was sure it wasn't what the neighbour told her about him being accused of inappropriate watching and words and then being asked, in a less than leisurely fashion, to abandon the pool for good.

It was, he told her, because he was focusing too much on his body and not enough on his soul and so he changed to Mr Zen, being present to each moment wanting simplicity and space. His new-found Buddhist leanings led him via tantra and the tedium of his endless, goalless, grinding, to celibacy, the only way to preserve his life force, his energy, his chi. She was relieved.

Mr Feng Shui Monk would spend hours talking to his miniature bonsais in koans, having set Beauty to work clearing, and emptying and throwing her old life away. He mocked her sentimental collecting of teenage mugs, her connection to old books and notes, her hoarding of her mother-bought coats, her stack of dog-eared teenage magazines and pouches of tangled chains and bangles. All signs of her lack of enlightenment. Her suffering, he told her, as he plunged her past into bin bags, was caused by her over-attachment to the material; there is no past, no future, just the present; she must work harder to let go, to be free. Of course he was right, she agreed, ignoring her breaking heart as she dropped her grandmother's hair brush into the gathering pile of detritus which had once been her precious sense of history and self.

No sooner than her former life was sent packing to the charity shops, or tip, or bin, did he revert to slovenly type, leaving cups to home-grow penicillin, adorning every chair and stair with his thrown-off dirty clothes and happily making his muddy mark across her newly wiped kitchen floor. The celibacy was banished by top-shelf magazines and soon he was back in the saddle, riding her hard. She complied, and silently mopped her crutch and then the floors.

His brooding, his sulking, was so powerful that it created a vortex, a vacuum sucking all the fun from life, all her sparkle, all her verve and vigour. She had spoken to him in the wrong tone, said it in the wrong way, used words he didn't like, hadn't answered his endless questions in the required way, hadn't told him enough detail about her day. She talked too much, asked too much, laughed too much. He didn't like noise, didn't like chatter, would roll his eyes when she talked to him, would flick through screens and fold his arms if ever she wanted to confide. Would turn his back or push her away if he'd had enough of what she was saying. He told her she was boring, that her opinions were stupid, uninformed, childish, misled. He didn't want to listen to what was of interest to her, had nothing of interest to say himself. And all of it was her fault. She was boring, irrational, irrelevant and wrong.

Even his screwing around was her fault. She had to be quiet about that too, it was none of her business, which is just as well as by now she had lost the words to say how hurt she was, how she felt betrayed. Beauty, feeling less beautiful by the day, pushed these things to the back of her mind, quietening her inner voice, her inner knowing was fading away. Delete, Delete, Delete. This isn't part of the story so let's just rub it all out. Delete. Anything to keep her fairy-tale story on track. Reframe, refocus, look at what's going well and ignore the rest.

And the rest of life was good. For when she stepped outside her double-glazed front door, designed to keep the noise out, the silencing incantation of her home lost its tenure, lost its twist, until returning she would insert the key to lock her voice once more away.

She loved work, where she grew and helped others grow. Standing up strong and energetic, shoulders back, smiling but concerned, she would radiate all that is comfort and warmth for the war-torn women who needed her help. The women who had to hide in shelters, who ran to escape their abuse, the women with their fag-burnt flesh, their kick-fractured bones, their missing teeth, their iron-marked skin. Sleeping Beauty would tend to them all, for they lived in a different dream from her, a nightmare, not of romance born, a different country, a different breed, not like her.

Not like her at all.

At all. As long as she was quiet and didn't say a word.

She did what good girls do; she tried harder, smiled more, shoved down her feelings, understood him more, made allowances, bent over backwards for him. She became a sexpert:

Tantric sex

Porn sex

Make-up sex

Calm-him-down sex

Cheer-him-up sex

Sex-so-he-doesn't-need-to-have-it-with-anyone-else sex

Sex-because-he's-had-it-with-someone-else sex

Reclaim-what-was-hers sex

Looking-for-security sex

Maybe-he'll-do-some-housework-after sex

Maybe-he'll-like-me-more sex

He-likes-it-when-I-dress-up sex

He-likes-it-in-front-of-a-mirror sex

If-I-don't-have-sex-he-calls-me-frigid sex

Who knew there were so many kinds of sex? Cosmo has really missed a trick not writing about these.

Hi-ho-hi-ho, it's on with the story we go, she smiles all day, she's fucked at night, hi-ho-hi-ho-hi-ho-hi-ho.

Let's watch her arrive home from work, bearing best-wishes-maternity flowers from much-loved and loving colleagues. Let's peep as she kicks off her shoes, wiggles her slightly swollen toes, and changes into more comfortable maternity clothes. She has left her job and she smiles secure in the knowledge that Heathcliff has work and will keep his family safe and fed.

No.

He quit work too.

Why should he keep working when she wasn't, that's hardly fair is it?

From Dinkies to Dolites. From double income, no kids, to no income with a new mouth soon to arrive.

Not good.

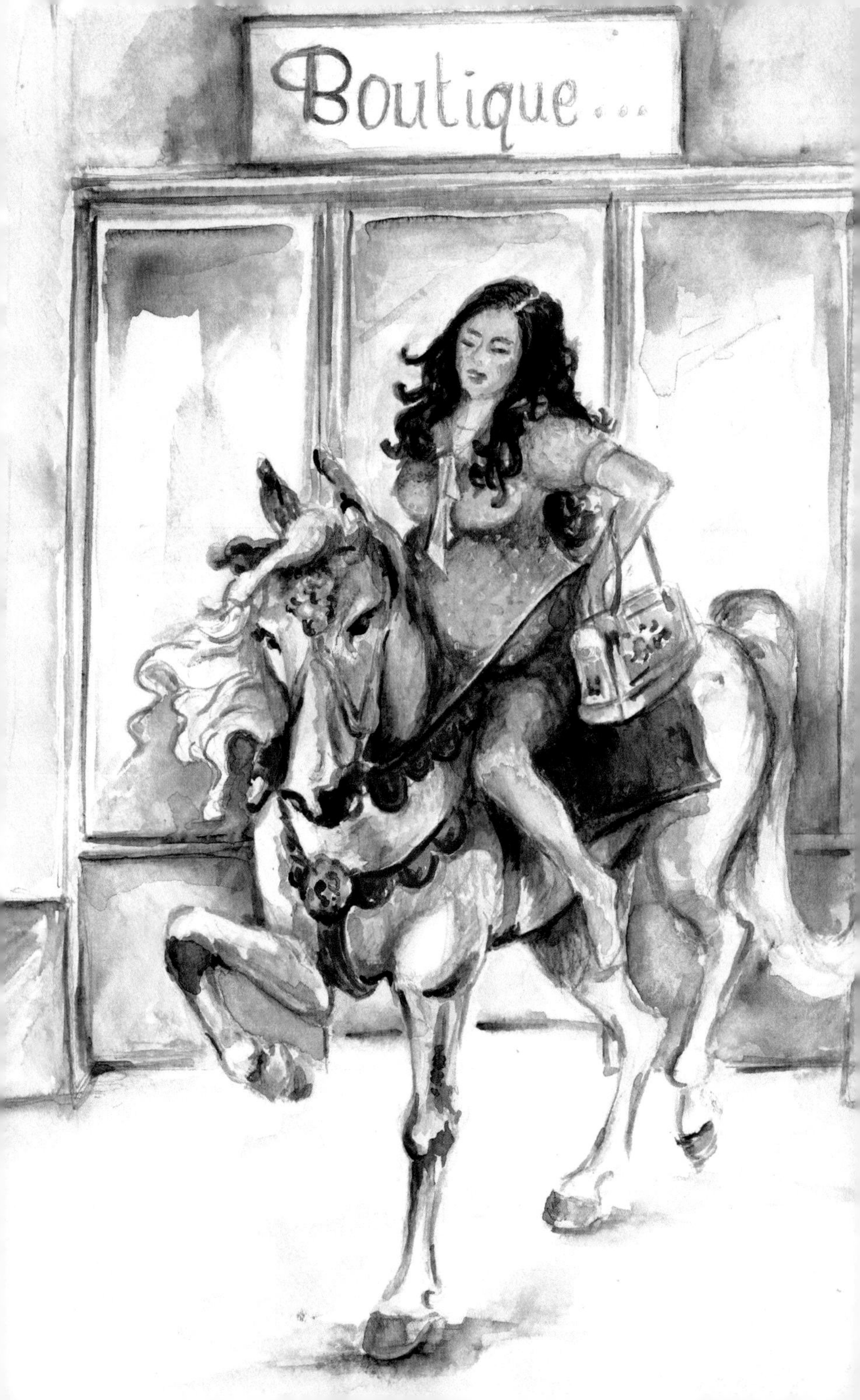
Boutique...

So she did what heroic-feminists do; summoned her white-charger, heaved herself back into the saddle and got another job, never letting her late-stage pregnancy slow her down. For she knew that all happy-ever-afters were built on dragons fought, rivers crossed, and that poverty was standard: Cinderella, Rose Red and Snow White. She worked until the day before the babe arrived.

Meanwhile poor Heathcliff got all depressed. Having a pregnant wife with her swollen teats and endless attempts at baby-name chatter, who could blame him? So, he went fishing. Often. In silence. Alone. Bliss.

She really was living the dream.

SO IT CAME TO PASS that Beauty went into labour and he, being the doting father-to-be that he was, got to the hospital a bit late, which was her fault, because she was inconsiderate enough to have started huffing and puffing just as he was about to land the biggest fish the world had ever seen. Her timing was always out, nothing to do with him.

Her contractions came thick and fast, wringing the life out of her womb and the strangled, primal ululations from her dry mouth. The tension rose, the baby was coming, drum roll...

Crash.

He'd hit the deck. Blacked out. Fainted. Heroic. As the nurses rush to his aid, mopping his brow, cradling his head against their warm and tender breasts, Beauty, apologetically, whispers; "I think I need to push. Er, could I have a little help please?"

Out cold, he missed the birth. But he made up for it with his first words about his newborn to his much-beloved wife; "I don't like babies."

Crack.

The sound of a heart breaking.

Crack.

The sound of a fragment of fairy tale falling to the linoed-hospital floor.

Crack.

A chink in the dreamy sleep of happy-ever-after, letting reality poke abruptly through.

Beauty was starting to wake up.

He didn't like his own son. Of course, he wasn't going to like this squalling-crying, screwed-up, snivelling babe; taking Beauty's attention away from him like that and giving nothing in return.

As his face contorted in jealousy and disgust, shock waves tremored across Beauty's tired and stretched skin. Armour started to weld around her heart. A fire of protective mother-love ignited, lion-like in its ferocity. No one would hurt her son. No one.

And he didn't.

At least not with fists.

Words and deeds were his weapons.

Rejecting the smooth-skinned chubby infant hand. Revolted by the runny nose, the smelly nappies, the suppurating birth wounds of the mother. Pushing away the growing-lively-lovely-wanting-a-cuddle toddler.

Mocking

Taunting

Insulting

Jeering

Jibing

Rejecting

Bullying

Ridiculing

Humiliating

Destroying the confidence of his own son. Daily. Hourly. Minute by minute. During every interaction.

Beauty tried her best to create a shield (a new type of sex: 'Sex-so-he's-nicer-to-our-son sex'), to challenge him, to show her son that what the father said was just not true. But Beauty's voice was weak and small and the father's poison leaked into the boy's pores and bones, weakening him, sapping his youth-blood, draining his spring, flattening his growth, clouding his joy.

Beauty knew she needed help, knew she needed elders, knew she needed a fairy godmother to help her out of this mess. She looked desperately around and found:

HER COLLEAGUES, who reminded her that she knew the theory, that she had the experience, that she had the contacts, that she could go on the courses, that it was down to her to work it out. Come on Beauty, back on your white charger and sort this dragon out, it's all down to you, you know. You're on your own.

HER WORK, with all those battered women; what was she making a fuss about when all Heathcliff did was moan and groan and spit out venom? He never bruised flesh, tore out hair, or made them eat their own shit. She was one of the lucky ones. What was she complaining about?

HER PARENTS, and their idyllic marriage, sugary sweet, pleasing people, keeping their heads down and weaving yarns of love conquering all, always. Their ideal marriage. Beauty, ashamed, had failed to live up to their dream. She wanted that for her son, wanted the happy-ever-after, mummy-loves-daddy, daddy-loves-mummy-and-his-darling-boy too. Don't we all?

For better, for worse
For richer, for poorer
In sickness and in health
To love and to cherish
Till death us do part

She had vowed and allowed worse, poorer and sickness; it was all part of the package bought in bulk from the church shelves.

The Church must know best. Her colleagues knew best. She clearly knew nothing.

And then Fate threw her a lifeline: he got a job. Just in time, it looked like the dream might still be possible.

Well, Fate can't actually take the credit, it was Beauty who got him the job. And a job that took him to another part of the land, away, leaving her alone with her son.

What a relief.

Life was so much easier for Beauty and boy. They laughed, they played, they tickled and giggled. They watched the swallows swoop and made jewels from dew drops and when daddy came home with love bites from other ladies, mummy turned a blind eye, determined she was not going to be another divorce statistic even though her so quiet, polite, Pollyanna-positive parents had finally spoken, finally dared to question whether enough was enough.

Enough was not enough. Instead Beauty sold up and moved to be with him, to keep the family together. Until death do us part.

Time for another baby. But this time she had no expectations. She didn't expect him at the birth. Birthing is women's work after all so Beauty should just get on with it.

So she did.

Again.

He hated this son too. Another pointless scrap of human life, making more mess and noise. No wonder he spent so much time outside the house.

Once upon a time, Beauty would have had witches, potion-makers, wise women, fairy godmothers to save her marriage, instead she could only find Family Therapy, which sadly lacked the power and potency to turn Frog-Heath into the prince of her dreams. Instead it just gave him more scope for mockery and ridicule.

But Beauty slumbered on with her good intentions and hope in her heart, not noticing the silencing of her boys, the way they scuttled, scrabbled, hushed and whispered, the way they turned inward, disappearing, whenever they heard their father's footsteps on the path.

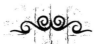

U NTIL ONE DAY, she travelled with her work, to see a modern-day magus, standing high and mighty on a stage. He summoned her forth, in front of the crowds, casting circles of power on the stage. He bid her stand in one circle she called 'Heath' and as always could see the world through his eyes, could see what he meant, what he needed, what he thought, what he said, what he wanted, how he judged, saw herself through his eyes, and saw how she had failed.

"Now," commanded the magus, "stand in circle number two, which is you."

"What? Me?"

Blank.

When she stood in her own circle she found that she could think of nothing; didn't know what she wanted, what she needed, what she liked, what she thought, what she felt. Nothing. She was invisible, transparent, only an echo of a person, a wisp, a shimmer, a whisper.

"Now," commanded the magus, "stand in circle three; the fully awake you, and tell me what you see."

Trepidation tingling, she tiptoed into the third vortex. The west wind of wisdom swirled up her legs, coiling up her torso and into her mind. The easterly wind of ego blew into her gut and woke her inner power. The southerly wind of self-love swept through her hair and down into her heart. The northerly wind of new-noticing opened her eyes wide and shook her to her bones.

Sleeping Beauty woke up.

Awake, alert, attentive at last, Beauty shook the scales of her dreams from her eyes and stood solidly in her own circle, her own power, and saw the truth of what she had never seen before.

She knew she had to leave.

With her new-found sword of truth, she eviscerated the romantic-princess and found, inside the silky-skin of pink-niceness, that she was taut and strong and smart. She slashed through his silken threads of threats and manipulation, she sliced through her procrastination, her compassion, her constant explanation and understanding and saw that he was poison. She ripped the silencing spell from its hinges and shrieked, banshee-wildness in proclamation at her new voice. She took her simpering-make-up-and-keep-the-boys-safe sex and dashed out its cowering. She chanted incantations, casting spells of separation, sending Heath back to the pond from whence he came. She stamped her feet and danced, drumming wildly to the beat of her heart around the sacred fire of self-love and power. Snarling at him when he came close, roaring, she clawed back her life and built a new den for her cubs to grow.

Finally, her sugar-plum parents spoke up loudly and helped out; better late than never, their support and understanding affirming her growth.

Her battles weren't over, Heath-Frog fought back using every trick and manipulation in his quiver.

He didn't answer the phone.

He didn't share the bills.

He blamed her and shamed her and named her to all who would listen.

He told her if he killed himself it would be all her fault.

He refused to leave the family home, she would have to find another.

He would phone and moan and blame and accuse and still Beauty's armour grew stronger.

She found a new house without the silencing spell at the door. Her home refilled with voices, play dates, girlfriends, workmates and family, made welcome in the chaos of her resettling, in the beauty of her unpacked boxes, in the glee of her happy boys.

T HE BOYS GREW UP to live their own stories. Beauty is still working, still healing. Here's what she would tell you, if you asked her what she'd learned, she'd share her voice and say;

"Although the dream is lovely, all shimmering and pink,
Get a grip and shake yourself awake, stretch your arms high and blink.
For the sleepers are enchanted, beguiled and entranced,
And then they are made to move to someone else's dance."

She would say;

"Wake up! Wake up! Take good care and don't hold back,
On asking for what you want and seeking what you lack.
Listen to your own thoughts first, trust your gut, find your morals,
For when you try to live for someone else it will only end in sorrow.'

Goldilocks and the three bears

ONCE UPON A TIME there was a girl with tangled, curling, caramel-honey hair.

Look at her first-day-at school photograph.

Nervous smile, eyes looking away from the camera, shoulders folding inwards over a second-hand school top. You can't see her bitten fingernails or her tense-white knuckles. This head and shoulder shot, brightly lit by silver umbrella and white screen, does not show her grass-stained knees and the mud which hides the scratches there etched. You cannot see the scuffs on her toes or the slime on the soles of her too-small, new-to-her, passed-down shoes. You can't smell her navy pants so don't notice the acid, nitrate smell of dried piss where she was frightened but there was no time to change, and even if there had been, she wouldn't have changed because wetting yourself got you a beating.

This photo doesn't show how humiliated she felt when she couldn't hold a pencil, when the other kids giggled at the squiggles on the page. No one saw how she was left alone at break, as the others moved away from her smell and gloom to skip and hop and play. She didn't know how to play and so sat and watched, from the corner of the yard, by the bins, curious at the gurgling, bubbling noises that she didn't recognise as laughter.

She loved her milk when the others crinkled their noses and yukked, she treasured this tiny vial of nurturing, just for her, new, untouched, not shared, not second hand, all her own. She was amazed at school dinners, unaware that the other children paid, she cleared every drop of viscous gravy, every mushed and mulchy pea, every soggy potato from her unchipped plate. At first too stunned and full to touch the jammy, fruity, sometimes chocolatey offerings that came to follow, she soon acquired a taste for gypsy tart; its smooth caramel, pristine until her spoon, clumsily held in unaccustomed fingers, marked it as her own.

The bosomed, aproned dinner lady watched with the eyes of one who has seen and known a thousand children come and go and saw how frail and pale this girl was, how silent and small. She noticed the twigs tangled in her golden curls, the dirt beneath her fingernails, the lice roller-coasting unattended behind her tendrilled ears. Yet when she spoke to the man who was in charge, he shrugged, barely looking up from his paperwork, another fussing woman and another dirty kid when he was doing spreadsheets and more important things.

So no one saw as Goldilocks left the gates at the home-time bell alone. No one saw how she scuttled in the shadows from the netball hoops and hopscotch, avoiding pavement cracks and black cats, through the town, where people were too busy with their shopping and their gossip to pay attention to a girl on her own, running, head down on skinny legs towards the wood.

NO ONE WATCHED as she pushed through the brambles even though they grabbed and tore her fair flesh; "All the better to hide us. We don't want nosey parkers coming here." No one saw as she ducked through the reaching branches and jumped the fallen, battered trunks; "All the better to put them off, we don't want them interfering with us."

No one saw as she arrived at the base of an old dark tree, how she knelt down, parted the ivy, pushed aside the sticks and lifted the mossy stones away. No one saw as she wiggled head first into a dark hole, no larger than it needed to be, and crawled down into the earth. She made herself invisible as she passed the spiders weaving their sticky webs, the maggots chewing on the fallen carcass of something that had once been a something, but what, she didn't know. Not even the centipedes paid attention to her passing, so silently she moved towards the higher cavern and the stone-rolled door. Here, no one saw her pause, glad to have circumvented her many legged neighbours, taking a breath before calling out that she was home.

Some days her mother would open the door, hair matted and greyed, clinging to her head for support, hands always shaking, feet flip-flopping unevenly along the earthen floor. These were the days Goldilocks liked best for it meant it was just her mother and she and for a time, whether a heartbeat, a breath or more, there was a tenderness that dare not other-times peek its head out of their hearts. They would hold hands, silently, skin to skin, both cracked and torn, both muddied and bloodied, one from the woodland thorns, one from mops and chopping and floors. When these moments stretched the mother would share a hidden treat, a blackberry saved, an acorn nestling in its cap, a feather dropped by a careless bird as it flew to feed its young. They would gaze together at the fragility and perfection, sniffing, tasting, caressing such beauty in such worn hands.

"Sunshine, you are my sunshine," her mother would sing softly with her long-forgotten voice as she held her girl child tightly to her bruised and aching chest, unable to remember the warmth of the sun on her scarred and pitted skin. They would inhale each other deeply; blood and earth, salt and stone mingling with flesh and bone to make them know each other's scented notes above all others. It seemed to Goldilocks that time had turned a blind eye for these brief moments of love and care, that it had napped or been distracted by a budding blossom or a fledgling's flight, for these moments were as pictures, bright and immortal, living in her memory where no one else could see, where they, if only they, were safe.

BUT TODAY was not such a day, for the stone was rolled away by the huge, black talons of her father's paw. Shrinking and dropping to all fours she scuttled past his legs of steel, his feet of lead, hoping that his tiny eyes ignore her, just this once. They never did, for Daddy Bear missed nothing, knew everything, saw all and ruled his land with a paw of bristles, sinew and strength. "Who's been lying on my bed and trampled all my fern?" he would bellow, ignoring that she slept on the hard floor alone. "Who's been sitting on my chair and smeared their scent on it?" he would roar, ignoring that he only let her sit on the packed mud floor. "Who's been eating my food?" he would demand, knowing that she couldn't reach the high hook where the meat was hung, and that all she was fed were the scraps spat out by father and son.

Hurling her across the cave of mud and wood, towards the smouldering fire he snarled at her to help her mother stoke the flames to cook their kill while he and Brother Bear relaxed and scratched and dozed as was only befitting of such powerful, handsome, fearsome beasts.

Brother Bear was a handful of years older than Goldilocks, much admired since birth, much desired by his father, a chip off the old block, that's my lad. Before he walked, he swaggered, before he could talk he could swear, before he could hug he hit, before he could ask he would demand and Mummy barely-there would run around and fetch and carry and cook and clean and do whatever it took to keep her male bears in the manner to which they soon grew accustomed. And when the mother barely-there found herself lumpen and swollen in spite of the belts and kicks, the Daddy Bear named the boy-baby inside her and gathered his mates for a celebratory drink of a second son.

The celebratory drink turned into a wake, a suffering, a commiserating; for out of the womb crept a wimpy, weedy girl child, not the expected thundering, mighty male. She struggled from her blood cave of warmth and pulsing into this veil of tears and knew no different to the beatings and shoutings her mother endured as she snivelled through her days. Goldilocks soon learned how to press cobwebs into her mother's cut flesh and make leaves into relieving poultices. Marigolds for healing, eye-bright for black eyes, fennel for when it hurt her mother to pee.

Goldilocks would hear muffles and gasping and sobbing at night and pull the moulded blanket further over her tangled, tousled head, blocking the sound with mildew and moths. When daylight lent its weak eye down the sooty chimney pot, Goldilocks tried not to see her mother dragging herself across the floor after her father's paw had melted her stomach. She tried not to see as her mother turned purple against the wall, eyes rolling back, white, as Daddy Bear's furry paw pushed hard against the soft skin of throat. She tried not to catch his eye in case he remembered her and saw her. She would turn herself invisible, blending in with the

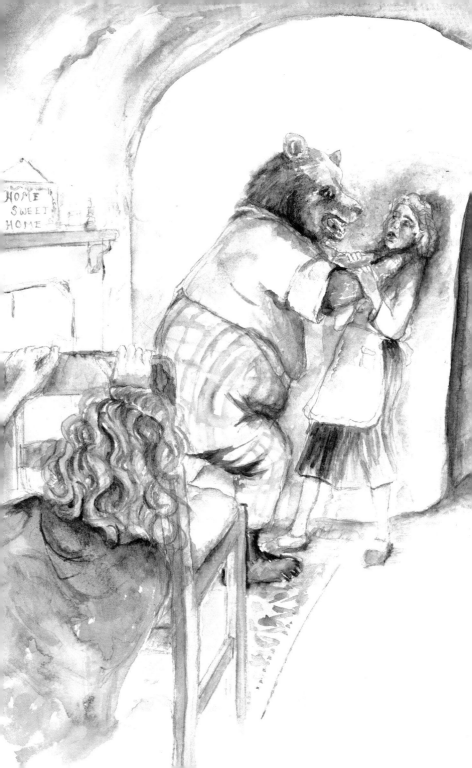

rough pots and pans, the brooms and blankets, blending in and holding her breath, eyes squeezed shut, hands over ears, if she couldn't see him, maybe he couldn't see her.

But Brother Bear saw her and tripped and nipped and punched and pulled and stole her food and hid her blanket and called her names she didn't understand. He would push her to the floor and push his meat-rotten snout into her pale speckled face, slavering and dribbling and watching her squirm. Goldilocks remembered the time Mummy Bear pulled Brother Bear off Goldilocks. She only did it once and for weeks, Goldilocks had to gather thistle down and feathers, moss and ferns to stem the blood which poured from between her mother's buckled legs.

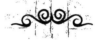

OW LOOK AT THIS PICTURE.
No it's not faded, the girl does indeed seem so pale in her junior school uniform, red cardigan paling her translucent, sun-forgotten skin. She's looking at the camera this time. Have you ever seen eyes so sad, so huge and grey with longing and loss? Her longer-tangle of twisting hair is dragged back from her fine boned face with an old elastic band, you can see her clavicle clearly empty, her shoulder bones jutting as they reach to touch across her chest. Her borrowed, lost-property blouse is hiding ribs like xylophones that play no melody, you would see her heart pushing again its cage, longing to be free.

This photo doesn't show her curly neat handwriting, practised quietly, alone, in the library, escaping the other kids and stares and jibes. Nor does it show the piles of books inside her head, consumed first in pictures, then in sounds and finally in words to waft her away from her here and now to places once upon a time and then. This picture doesn't show her ease with numbers, their logic clear and precise, knowable and true, her love of prediction and accuracy, her chewed pencil and her rubbings out.

This picture doesn't show Miss White who looks at Goldilocks and sees beyond the still-scuffed shoes and muddied knees to the brain that ticks and turns with agility and speed. You would not see Miss White sneaking new pens and pencils into Goldilocks grateful still-chewed hands. You can't see the extra portions of lunch Miss White ensured the ladles served, the only food her shrivelled stomach sometimes had. This picture doesn't show the moments Miss White spends with this small tangled girl, trying to straighten her out, to stick plasters on her knees, to see if she can get her to tell her the story of her home. Nor would you see the telephone calls leading nowhere to try and get Goldilocks some help.

One day Goldilocks arrived at school before dawn and pushed herself into the corner by the door to wait for Miss White. Miss White arrived, armed with books and bags and was almost through the door before the waif raised herself and wafted in. "Please Miss, my mum needs help." And so the words explained, as best they could without the understanding to make it clear, how Mummy Bear was getting fat, really fat, with a big lump that stuck out in front and made Mummy Bear waddle and hold her back. How the bump made it hard for Mummy Bear to bend and to fetch and to carry. How Daddy Bear seemed even more cross with Mummy Bear because she couldn't do the work she had to do and how he couldn't lie on top of her at night and make the snuffling sounds because the bump got in the way.

The words wove from a mouth too small to tell of the kicking which first started in her mother's legs, sending her toppling over to her knees. The words winced to tell of how the bear foot crashed into the Mummy Bear's back over and over even when she begged for mercy, begged for it to stop. The words cried as they told of Daddy Bear sat on Mummy Bear's bump and bounced around while his paws sliced and scored across Mummy Bear's face. The words couldn't even begin to explain what Daddy Bear did with his pee-pee between Mummy Bear's legs whilst the daylight closed its eyes and looked away. The words managed to utter the unthinkable; that Mummy Bear was lying mewling in the den with blood coming out from between her legs and Goldilocks couldn't clean the blood away, and it was sticky, and there had never been so much before and Mummy Bear asked Goldilocks to get some help quick, please quick.

So help was called and blue lights trampled the forest floor and found the hole and dug the Mummy Bear out, covered in twigs and leaves, dropping, dripping, whimpering and holding her tummy tight.

Mummy Bear went to the big white building with lots of white people with lots of long wires and funny smells and where the ladies with the aprons smiled at Goldilocks with sad eyes and made her extra hot chocolate and toast with a wink.

Mummy Bear stopped bleeding but she didn't stop crying and the bump from her tummy was gone leaving a wobbly, jellied mess which swung away from her when she leaned this way or that. Goldilocks was looked after by a lady like Miss White, someone who was clean and smiling and kind and who had soft white things to sleep on and silver things to carry food to your mouth. Goldilocks asked where Daddy Bear was and where Brother Bear were, but no one seemed to know, not even Mummy Bear who didn't seem to be able to speak words which could be understood anymore.

Then men in blue went to see Mummy Bear and Goldilocks had to leave the quiet, white room and went with the kind ladies to a room filled with yellow and orange and blue and red sharp shapes that she didn't know what to do with until the lady showed her how to stick them together to make a rainbow wall. Goldilocks saw the men in blue shrug their shoulders and shake their heads as they left Mummy Bear's room. Goldilocks didn't understand what the clean white ladies said to Mummy Bear about how she should press charges. Goldilocks saw Mummy Bear turn her face to the wall.

Then Mummy Bear left the white bed and Goldilocks left the silver food things and they went back to a different den, a darker den, further into the woods. She had to wiggle past the goblins polishing and gloating their stolen treasure troves. Lying low Goldilocks and Mummy Bear dragged themselves, reaching hands forward to pull themselves on their bellies past the upturned vampires, dripping blood, awaiting nightfall for their erotic, bloody, play to the dark iron door of their new home. They had no key but the bolts rammed home and the door swung open.

Daddy Bear was angry with Goldilocks for telling the teacher. Daddy Bear was cross with Mummy Bear for telling Goldilocks to get help. Brother Bear laughed as Daddy Bear taught them a lesson.

Goldilocks moved schools.

Goldilocks never told anyone anything again.

HERE'S ANOTHER PICTURE.

No, it's not the light. Goldilocks has faded even more. Look closely and you can see a ghostly outline of where she used to be. See how her hair is cobweb white-blond and her skin is fingernail grey, see her eyes look far and away. See her in her new uniform, the black jumper helping her fade to grey, allowing her to blend in with the crowd of other heavily bagged secondary school children, holding their planners to ward them off from detentions and getting lost. She's on all the registers but no one knows who she is, she keeps her head down, keeps silent, keeps herself to herself.

She hates PE, she tries to disappear into the gossip to hide her jutting ribs where the other girls have breasts blooming. Sometimes she worries that they will see the bruises and the burns, but they are all too busy with chatter of first leg-shaving and sanitary products to notice one as insubstantial as she.

The bells made her jump, make her heart pound, her hands shake. When the teachers shout - though never at her, for to shout at her would mean they had noticed her and they never did - she would duck and wince, shoulders up around her ears, eyes squeezed shut, trying to wish it all over, all away. She does her work on time, quickly, neatly, never giving the teachers a reason to notice her.

Break time knew she hid in the library, lunchtime knew she did too, the library watched as she read and wrote and calculated and underlined work to hand in so she didn't have to take it home. She couldn't take it home.

The dinner ladies didn't notice her, the free school dinner form was burned by Brother Bear to keep her in her place. She was in her place. Brother Bear and Daddy Bear made sure she knew that.

Since the white room, Mummy Bear was silent. There were no more smiles or hand holding, she never looked up even though they toiled together to keep the male Bears fed and kept. Neither watched as the other's beatings were borne. There was nothing that could be done. No point in crying, that just makes it worse, gives them more energy to go on longer. Just hope it passes soon. Or that it all goes black. It sometimes does.

SEE THIS PICTURE:

Yes indeed she does still look so young, so fragile, so pale. Yes, she's still at school but there is no uniform in the sixth form. She wishes there was. She stands out more now with her borrowed, charity clothes amongst the labels and the makeup, the trainers and the bags. It's not exactly bullying, if you asked her she would shrug, names are nothing, sticks and stones do break your bones and names can no longer hurt her. Some teachers know her now. She surprised them and herself with the grades that came in the summer. Who'd have thought? No one even knew who she was and yet she had clearly been there, a diamond in the rough. Odd but bright.

The library and she were old friends, it saved her desk, kept her safe, kept her away from the peering and the glances, away from the whispers as she walks to lessons alone. The library lends her the books the other students own and gives her paper and pens too. There is even a special space where she can leave her things, where they are secure. Her physics teacher sees her work hard and late, sees that she doesn't go home when the other kids do, notices that she never seems to eat. He asks her how she is, is she OK? She nods and politely says thank you, then returns to her books.

She's working after school, sweeping up other people's hair, sterilizing combs, making tea, all invisibly. Janine tells her she has lovely hair, so pale, so fine. Her curls have gone, without straighteners, her hair too tired and scared to curl. Janine talks a lot and Goldilocks is good at listening and at the end of the week Goldilocks takes her small brown envelope, unopened, back to the den.

Janine asks her about school. Goldilocks says it's OK and then Janine goes on at length about the teachers she hated and the detentions she had. Janine asks her about parties and Goldilocks says she doesn't go and doesn't add that no one invites her and then Janine regales her with tails of spin the bottle and vomit. Janine asks her about boyfriends and sex and Goldilocks blushes and shrugs and cannot match what happens to her at home with Janine's juicy tales. Goldilocks knows what rape means now. And incest. Her periods have never started. She is glad. She is glad Janine talks a lot. She likes Janine.

Janine likes Goldilocks. God she works hard, never seen anyone get the sinks so clean, not a hair out of place, like she's had years of practice. She never complains, is never late, is always deferential. A bit too deferential now she came to think about it, she needed bringing out of her shell. So skinny too. Too skinny. Janine wants to feed her. Goldilocks doesn't want food. Doesn't want curves. Wants to be invisible. It's getting harder to remain unseen.

At school the sessions start on how to apply for university or get an apprenticeship or leave home. Her three science teachers rave about her grades, about her prospects, about how there needs to be more women in science, about what a great brain she has. She doesn't tell them that science is safe, there is cause and effect, there are logical patterns, evidence to support statements, precision and order, objectivity and ethics. Science allows for prediction, estimation, categorization, it makes meaning out of chaos. She can not leave home. She will not leave home. She can not leave her mother.

Her mother, whose teeth are black or gone, whose back is buckled, whose legs are swollen and twisted, whose dead eyes see only the floor. Goldilocks needs to be there for her mother, has to help, has to get the food on the table in time, cooked well. Has to sweep the floors, has to scrub clothes and shoes and the toilet pot. It's the only way to keep her mother safe. And yes, she sometimes has to shut her eyes and endure the snuffling, gasping weight of bear flesh, dreaming that she is far away, distanced from her body, mind soaring far away.

Janine notices something odd some days, sees that Goldilocks scrubs her hands until they bleed, sees the ever-present eczema raise and purple. Janine notices that some days Goldilocks is even more nervous than others, that the bell announcing clientele makes her wince and quiver. She sees that some days Goldilocks can hardly get her breath, her chest seems to heave as if it would break, as if her heart is leaping to escape. Never shy Janine has asked about PMT, about rows at home, about boyfriend trouble and is starting to notice that she can't get any answers, no clues, no patterns. Janine hates a mystery. She's a hairdresser, they know everything about everyone but never pass on gossip, although she'd love to, but it's really bad for business.

Janine is pleased that Goldilocks isn't going to university, all that debt and what's the point when you can work here and I'll teach you how to wash hair. So Goldilocks is promoted and finds herself tilting heads back with suds and towels and the customers hardly notice the hands that massage their care worn skulls as they spew their lives aloud cloaked in a nylon cutting gown. Goldilocks is stronger than she looks. They like her massage. They leave her tips. The tips don't go into the small, brown envelope. Goldilocks is confused and panicked. Janine can't work out why but tells her to keep them in an empty tea caddy that's ugly but a customer gave it to her so she can't give it away.

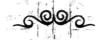

LOOK AT THIS PHOTO:
This is the one Janine insisted on, the salon staff (she and Goldilocks and Emma who works on a Saturday and a half day in the week). Lime green tabards with black T-shirts and leggings, which Goldilocks bought with her tips. She had never bought new clothes before. Didn't know where to start so Janine took her in hand and took her out at the end of a long quiet day to guide her through the trying on and tills, confused at this ingénue. They had even giggled together when Goldilocks had to buy children's clothes, cheaper at least. She'd never seen Goldilocks giggle before, she put her hand over her mouth as if trying to hold it in. She was actually pretty Janine noticed, surprised.

There is a man who comes in every third Tuesday, on market day, smelling slightly of shit and hay. He takes off his cap and winks at Janine and Goldilocks before submitting to Janine's snipping. He starts to have his hair washed first. Janine teases him, calls him posh, nudges Goldilocks who finds herself feeling uncomfortably hot. He is loud and laughs like a horse. His hands have ground-in dirt on them. His shirts are always spotless and his brown boots too. He has a bald patch on the top of his head which he denies and Janine threatens to use her shiny phone to provide photographic evidence. He laughs easily. He is big. Wide. Tall. His name is Bob. His mother calls him

Robert. He goes quiet and mmms a little when Goldilocks washes his hair. He compliments her on her massage. He likes firm hands. I bet you do winks Janine. Goldilocks curls up inside and wants to float away like a soap bubble.

Janine says it is time for Goldilocks to learn to cut hair and pays for her to go to college one day a week to learn. Goldilocks is terrified that there will be less in the small brown envelope she takes home so she adds in the coins from the tea caddy (which Janine makes sure make up the difference, even when they don't). And so it is that now Goldilocks is trimming split ends, sticking pins in curlers on thinning, still proud heads, trying not to nip the ears of the wiggling school kids, bribed by their parents who want them tidied up. And she cuts Bob's hair now. She knows at first, that she is not very good but he is kind, he is patient, he makes her smile. He tells her she is pretty and likes to see the colour rush to her pallid throat. She starts to notice the small curls at the nape of his neck. He has a dimple in his left cheek. He wears a big scratched old watch with a curling leather strap. His father's watch he tells her when she comments.

She listens and she learns about the price of pork, the Ministry of Agriculture, the National Farmers' Union. She knows about his four brothers, his two sisters, his mum and dad who have known each other from birth, who have farmed since they could walk. She knows all about his first sow, the litter, the slaughter house. She knows how he left school as soon as he could, all those pointless books. She hears about how he was feeding as soon as he could toddle, herding when he could barely be seen over the sow's broad back. She knows how hard it is to walk through thick, black mud on a sodden autumn day when your short arms are struggling to carry the feed without spilling it. She listens well and likes that he doesn't ask about her. She doesn't need to talk.

Janine watches and smiles and isn't at all surprised when he asks Goldilocks out for a cup of tea and a slice of cake in her lunchtime. Of course, that's fine, she nods ignoring Goldilocks' panic and opening the door. NoNoNoNoNoNo thinks Goldilocks, what if someone sees, if her father or brother hear of it. But she has no choice, it feels, but to go and she rather enjoys the sweet hot tea in flowered, fluted cups, on tiny fragile saucers, she has never known such delicacy. He tells her more about waking at dawn, about Young Farmers japes and jests, about the bats under the eaves and the rats in the barns with the constantly breeding cats. She listens and finds she likes that he has chosen her to tell, so earnestly, the details of his life.

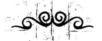

LOOK AT THIS PHOTOGRAPH:

It was taken on Janine's phone, she caught them holding hands as they came along the ordinary street towards her salon door. The sun blurs it but still you can see a pale, sylph of a woman, her hand lost in the giant paw of a man in khaki. She is looking up at him. He is looking ahead. They are at a distance so you cannot see the detail of their faces but you see her stride slightly behind his, her arm stretched to keep up with his long stance. The door frame of the salon cuts across the left hand corner, hardly the perfect shot but one which made Goldilocks blush when Janine showed her as they closed up that night.

Then here's another he insisted on.

No sunshine now, the winter has arrived. He's wrapped up in wax jacket and woollens and Goldilocks is wrapping her arms around herself for warmth, as he wraps his arms around her, standing tall behind her, towering. He is beaming with his prize, she looks like a startled hare, snared, but unsure that there isn't some comfort there. She allowed herself to lean back into his solid, warm, form and finds that there is support for her there. Her shoulders relaxed from up around her ears.

Janine is no longer surprised when Bob is waiting at the door for Goldilocks at closing time. She notes, with pleasure, that the afternoon tea that led to suppers is causing Goldilocks to curve, her hair to re-curl. She watches as Bob talks and Goldilocks listens but beneath the teasing smiles and snatched photos, she notices that there is something not quite right.

"Does he ever ask about you?" she asked one day as they folded towels behind the closed sign on the slightly smeared door. Goldilocks just shrugged and smiled and turned away with a "What's to say?" He didn't need to know about her now-incontinent mother whose balance was her enemy, always tripping her up. He didn't need to know that Goldilocks rose at the crack of dawn to scrub and wash and cook and slave so that her mother didn't have to. How could she tell him about the blood-stained sheets on her parent's marital bed? He must never know about her father's nocturnal visitations. Never know. Never.

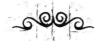

SEE THIS PHOTOGRAPH: This is the one taken on the second Christmas after the first slice of cake. His mother took it on the instamatic, why are they always kind of purple? That's Bob's father, his four brothers stand behind. Goldilocks is in her usual position, in front of Bob, encircled from behind by his strong arms, with his sisters on either side. They are standing in front of the old dresser, loaded with matching crockery, its edges gilded with worn-off gold. There is one small boy, his hair combed flat, the only grandchild. "That's odd." Janine had said, "Why is only one of them married? Why is there only one grandchild?" It didn't add up, that all but the married sister were still living at home.

Goldilocks shrugged and said she liked the close, loud, bustle by stove and yard and pantry. She liked how the sisters cooked and the brothers drove the tractors and the diggers, turning the wheels one handed, with their loyal dogs by their side. There was always a fire in the grate and the mother and father would sit side by side, holding hands, after decades of marriage and kids. The yellow sandstone walls seemed so warm and solid, so bright and calm, so different to the dark walls of the den, with its cobwebbed decorations and the hallway of night creatures snickering as she passed.

There was no wedding photograph.

Janine was furious. What had she worn? Who went? Who were the guests? Why hadn't she been invited or told? Did she wear white? Let's see the ring. Are you sure you've done the right thing? Goldilocks shrugged and explained that they hadn't wanted a fuss. That they had nipped out to the registry office, quietly. They used the official witnesses, men in dark suits, one with a pen behind his ear who kept checking his watch and tutting. Her family were not there. Of course. How could she tell her mother?

Bob took this next photo:

He hadn't wanted to, didn't see why Janine was making such a fuss about having one. It was natural that Goldilocks would give up work now she was his wife, she'd be helping on the farm instead. Janine's bright red hair, scrapped back in a high ponytail, face painted with contouring and colour which doesn't hide her sadness and concern. She loves this girl, as she would a younger sister. It's been nearly a decade now since an awkward school girl had come asking for work. Janine realises how little she knows about her sister-employee. Doesn't know where she lives, nor anything about her family. She seems to remember that she did alright at school, could have gone to university. Now she wonders whether she should have. Janine has her arm around Goldilocks' waist. Goldilocks is twiddling her wedding ring, leaning in and at the same time moving away.

There are no photos of the moment when Goldilocks tells her mother she is married and that she is leaving.

There doesn't need to be; the image of her mother's crumpled face will stay with her forever. She asks Bob to come with her when she tells her father and brother. It turns out Bob knows them, from the pubs, but hadn't made the connection, hadn't realised the Bears had a daughter at all.

There are no pictures of the back slapping and the hand shaking or the hissed; "Good riddance" of a wedding blessing from her father and the words of prophesy from her brother "You'll be just like our mother now."

There are no pictures of the wedding night where Bob is too hurried to notice the entrance way is already clear.

There are no photos of the room in his parents' house they have to call home.

There are no photos of Goldilocks scrubbing pots and pans, hauling pails through winter mud.

There is nothing to show of the mountains of ironing she daily clears, the dogs she feeds, the cats she tries to catch and worm. When Bob is away at market, she takes orders from the other men, do this, go there, do it faster, work harder. The brothers are hard workers, quick thinkers and she can't keep up with their expectations, she disappoints them.

There are no pictures to show how her muscles grow, how her skin hardens, how her pale bear-den face takes on a ruddy hew from the all-weather working.

Goldilocks doesn't question that the men eat first, whilst the women, having cooked, carry on with the outside feeding, then return to eat what is left. There is usually something left. The sister who lives at home is a good cook, the mother too. Goldilocks is not. She has so much to learn and had better learn it quickly too. They have sharp tongues to encourage her.

Goldilocks doesn't think it odd that after dinner the men sit down to watch TV and smoke whilst she and the mother tidy up and lay the table for breakfast, before polishing boots and wiping down overalls and putting the final wash on to hang up at dawn. When Bob takes her hand and leads her up the narrow stairs to bed, she is so tired she can hardly walk and is glad when, having mounted her, he is quickly spent. They are both asleep in an instant.

She doesn't notice when the brothers call her dim-witted and slow. When the father orders her to bring his lunch. When the mother bosses her in the kitchen. When the sister mocks her ironing. She doesn't question that she has no money of her own, that everything she has belongs to the family, that Bob buys all her clothes. She is used to getting up at dawn and working until dusk and beyond. She is used to her eczema flaring and being cold. She has no idea that she can say no to Bob at night, it never crosses her mind. All she knows is that here the only things that get kicked or hit or beaten are the beasts. Only the kittens are suffocated. She has forgotten that she used to like science, that the teachers begged her to go and study more. She has forgotten the laugh she had with Janine, her kindness, her care and her harmless, almost discrete gossip.

She never forgets her mother. At first Bob allowed her to visit on a Sunday when she would cook and clean and scrub the den and stroke her mother's balding head as she snuffled. But then there was just too much work to do on the farm and she could go next week, then the next and then next week never came and Goldilocks couldn't drive and had no money for a cab, so she knuckled down and got on with slopping out or loading up or whatever she was told to do.

There was no lens to catch the moment when she bumps into Janine on the street. Luckily there is no evidence of the shock and distress on Janine's face as she sees Goldilocks straggling, thinning hair, hunched shoulders, twisting, blistered fingers and black bagged eyes. No one saw the hasty hug or the whisper of concern followed by "Come back and work for me. I'm opening a bigger salon in a town further afield, there's a flat in the eaves, you could have it. Come and work with me."

There is no other answer but "No."

F YOU LOOK carefully at this blurry black and white image, crossed with the wires of scans, you can see the head here, the toes curled there and it seems to be sucking its thumb. Too young to tell the sex yet. Heart pumping, four cavities expanding and contracting in harmony. The twelve week scan. "How could you not know?"

"Because I so rarely bled," Goldilocks wanted to say, "only a speck here, a spot there. I could never be sure it wasn't when he'd been a bit rougher than usual when the lights were out." Of course she'd had the talks at school and listened to the other girls gossip and compare notes on pads or tampons. But it had never seemed relevant to her; so little did. Her life had been so different then, in the den with Daddy Bear and Mummy Bear and Brother Bear, so unlike the girls with tampons up their sleeves as they went in pairs to the old school loos.

"Get rid of it!" said Bob. "We don't need another mouth to feed, there's too much work to do. I thought you'd taken care of things." So Bob took her to the clinic and waited for her while the tiny life was sucked away. She was too young to be sterilized so the coil was the next best thing, no mistakes then. She doesn't remember if it hurt. She was numb. Just nothing. Floating above her body from afar, looking down, wanting to drift away on a rainbow bubble of light.

And as she floated on high, watching the men in white between her legs she remembered other silver things, another woman on another bed, with blood reddening the sheets. As she looked down she saw what she hadn't seen before, that Bob was a bear too. A different bear, not one with sharp claws, but one with sharp words and teeth, one who owned and caged her.

She knows she has to go. 'You'll end up just like our mother' the words taunting her. No. No. NoNoNoNo.

So she worked hard and did what she was told and didn't wince at night and never answered back. The months passed. The nights drew in and then exhaled again. One day he takes her into market with her, trusting her with a list of things to do; cheques to pay in, tools to sharpen, vet bills to pay. "Be back here by one." She is. As she rushes from one errand to another, her eyes are scanning, she's not sure for what, she's looking for a sign. There is none.

Market days become regular. She remembers how she met him in the salon when he came in for his trim. There is a tattoo parlour there now. Things have moved on. She doesn't recognise her face in the window as she passes, instead she sees her mum. Her mum. She hears no news of her mum and fears the worse. She has no way of knowing.

The years come and go and her hair streaks white from gold. Her belly is rock hard with muscle earned from dragging bales around the yard. She still knows she has to go but she has no money of her own and she can't go home.

HERE IS THE PICTURE that makes a difference. The one that changed everything. On the front page of the local paper is Janine, as if time had stood still for her, red ponytail high and bright on her head, Goldilocks would know her anywhere. A chain of salons. Award winning. Gala opening a great success, bringing business to the town. A further town. A bigger town. She knows where. She knows which road. A plan forms.

Goldilocks starts to run around the farm, her energy impresses them, at last she's shaping up. Her jobs done in half the time, now she's fencing and clearing ditches too. She has even learned to drive a tractor. Not a bad investment brother Bob, a good piece of stock she is.

She needs to wait until the spring fayre, the market day is longer as all the hill farmers bring their stock to the pen and ring. She is trusted now about the town, even given a couple of quid to buy a butty for lunch, a treat after all these years.

The day arrives. As he heads off towards the ring, she pockets the list of things to do, and hides the things she is meant to carry to repair or return and heads north, head down, remembering her skill learned from school, of turning herself invisible again.

Once she is past the peeping blinds and the nattering lawns, she starts to trot, picking up speed as the road divides, watching the signs and feeling the rhythm of her toned, strong legs.

Thoughts pester as she runs. What if he finds her? What if someone sees her? What if the salon is shut? What if Janine doesn't remember her? What if she won't help? All the time she has to bring her attention back to her feet on tarmac, oblivious to the curious glances of the passing drivers at this middle-aged woman running with ease in an old grey skirt and out-of-date trainers.

Running feels good. She feels strong and free. For the first time in charge of her own destiny. She smiles at the birds in acknowledgement of shared experience. The further town approaches, her heart hammers louder. She realises she has no idea where the salon is. She will have to ask. She has an hour before he will miss her. She needs to have vanished by then. She sees a school girl, chewing gum and kicking stones and asks her, and of course she knows, its where the school girls get their hair-ups for the prom.

The huge silver glass windows see her coming before she sees them and smirk at her reflection, not their usual clientele. "Is Janine here?" she asks. "I'm a friend of Janine's."

Hesitation. More smirking. Shared glances of amusement among the oh so young and cool in black pierced staff. "It's her day off," shrugs one. Goldilocks' knees go weak, she wobbles and has to sit. They don't like the idea of her sitting there for long, putting off clients. "She's upstairs, doing the books. I'll see if she's free," says one taking pity.

It seems the clock has stopped. The air is still. Goldilocks cannot breathe. She finds herself floating in a bubble looking down at a woman just like her mother, stooped and hopeless and old out of place on the mauve, velvet chair.

Janine sees her. Understands at once and without words, glares at the staff to get back to their work before taking Goldilocks by the hand and leading her upstairs. And so it is that the tears came. The tears are tidal, welling up from the infant years, gathering momentum as they rise as waves through puberty and beyond. There is no photograph of that first hour, of Janine's silent holding on as Goldilocks rides out the storm of all her loses and all her pain. No one saw as Janine stroked the care worn brow until Goldilocks fell asleep and then covered her with a blanket and then cried herself that there was such cruelty in the world. No one saw two women leave long after salon closing time, and drive to a modest house, where Janine held the key and made a bed and let Goldilocks rest.

THIS IS THE PICTURE that one of the cool, black-pierced stylists showed her mates. It captures a family of farming bears shouting and growling in the salon. It can't show how they were demanding that Janine return their goods, a wife, nor the shrug that Janine gave before picking up the phone to call the police. The stylist told her friends how scared she was, how she took the picture as evidence, from behind the stock room door, just in case anyone was hurt. No one was hurt.

But here is the picture the local paper took the next day of the broken salon window and the "slag" scrawled in red across the plated door held together with police tape telling others to keep out. The picture can not show the smell of bear piss on the upturned salon chairs and the pig shit trodden through the lino floor. They didn't take photos of the mixed hair dyes smearing threats along the wall or the scissors stabbed into the purple, velvet sofa where they didn't know but guessed that Goldilocks had sat.

Here is the police photo of Bob the Bear, apprehended just as he was about to pour petrol through a modest suburban door where two women had escaped through the back gate and over the garden wall.

Here is a headline photo of the bears as they are leaving court having watched Bob the Bear sentenced and sent down and ordered to pay damages to a certain hair salon in town.

Look at this photograph of Janine and her team, standing proud, outside the newly glazed salon, with the sun bouncing off the glass making Janine's high red ponytail sparkle in the light. Business is booming. No one ever liked the bears and Janine had conducted herself with such dignity through such a hard time that people were happy to put their hair in her team's hands.

There is no photograph to show how Goldilocks returned to her childhood den, many moons after her escape, to try to bring her mother out with her. Janine and friends had kept look out to warn in case Daddy and Brother Bear returned, phones ready to dial 999 should trouble brew. But there was no trouble, only more tears for Mummy Bear who wouldn't leave her pit, was too scared that there would be worse outside the den. Goldilocks never saw her again.

HERE IS THE PHOTO a passer-by took of Janine and Goldilocks waiting in the departure lounge, arms wrapped around each other, eyes full of tears and Goldilocks clutching a letter of recommendation to a salon-owning friend of Janine's away from all the trouble and bears. Janine never changes, her hair is still red and high, her cheekbones contoured and controlled, her neat black slacks and painted nails, she is timeless. Goldilocks is fit and strong from running miles across hills each day, trying to escape the bears that live on in her head, making her jump, stealing into her dreams, worrying her every thought and hope.

She can never outrun them.

HERE IS THE PHOTO that Janine received, airmail, of the salon team in the far-off land and there is Goldilocks at the back, looking browner, hair the colour of gold-white sand. She is still strong, still haunted, still running along the beach hoping the head-bears will drown and leave her alone so she no longer has to be so afraid, so alone, so mistrusting.

They never leave her alone.

Here is the photo that Janine is most proud of, Goldilocks with whitening curls, holding her graduation scroll which, the letter says, has been quickly followed up by a teaching post. It is never too late it seems, to make a fresh start.

Here is the staff badge with Mrs G Locks, Teacher of Science pictured, sternly in black and white. The kids think she is old and whisper about her behind her back, some things never change she thinks, knowing she looks older than she is. Knowing she could outrun even the fittest kid. Knowing that even though the bears still chase her in her sleep and make her heart beat at loud noises and shouting, she can breathe herself calmer. Knowing the bears will never go away but that life carries on anyway.

Rapunzel

NOT SO LONG AGO, nor so far away, there lived a large family in the twinkling, blarney, Emerald Isle. They loved their God and their prayers; loved their rosaries and their children; which is just as well as there were seven of them. The Pope would be pleased.

There was Majella, Madeleine, Aloysius, Camillus, Phelim, Alfonsius and Rapunzel. Don't worry too much about who was the oldest or the smartest of the toughest or the kindest, there were too many for the mother to keep tabs on, so what chance do we stand?

Anyway, there they all were, around the scrubbed wooden table, knees knocking, heads bowed, elbows budging, hands praying and gracing the food on the table;

Bless us oh Lord
And these your gifts
We praise you for saving us
Help us give you glory every day
Through Jesus Christ our lord
Amen

Amen for the scorching, mother-made broth, for the rough-cut bread, for the chipped white plates saved from Co-op stamps, for the family.

Amen for the mother shouting orders to the sisters, do that, do this, mend this, make that, go here, go there, like this, like that.

Amen for the quiet, hiding-behind-his-paper father.
Hail Mary full of Grace
Blessed are the women
And blessed are the fruits of their wombs

Amen for the girls of the house doing the washing up, the cleaning, the ironing, the stitching and mending, the scrubbing, the caring.

Amen that the boys could just sod off outside and play.

Joy.

And yet there were moments of not quite joy, but glee. Moments of snickering and suppressed giggles, behind scrubbed hands with mouths squeezed shut and eyes brimming with mirth as the seven parodied their zealous, devout mother at prayer. There was a warmth in the teasing, a connection in naughtiness, the only true place that feelings flowed; in this sinful, collusion of mockery.

Honour your father and mother that your days may be long
Children obey your parents in the Lord for this is right

Naughty, naughty boys and girls, three Hail Marys and confession for you.

There was no time for feelings, too much washing and cooking to do. These were the days before microwaves and automatic washing machines; you modern women don't know you're born!

These poor emotionally banished children of Eve sent their sighs and mourning and weeping inward, locked them down deep in their hearts and souls. For man (and woman, so they are taught, must learn self-mastery and domination of emotion in order to find peace..

They expected nothing more than a vale of tears in this life, and knew, for sure, their reward, if they followed the rules, to a T, would be in heaven.

It would have been more than a vale of tears if the boys' crusted socks had ever been discovered under the sheets, for we all know that if a man allows himself to be governed by his passions, he loses his dignity and becomes unhappy. Masturbation is an intrinsically and gravely disordered action. Amen. A-men. Ah-men to that.

Shame it felt so good.

Forgive me father for I have sinned.

Again.

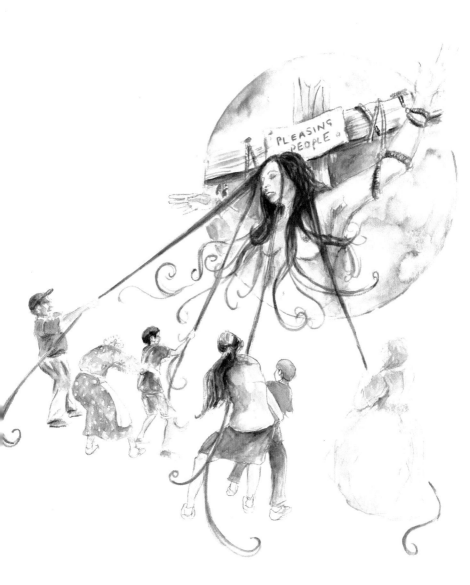

Hail Mary.

As for the girls, well, no need to worry about them, luckily, they knew that chastity was a moral virtue, a gift from God, and so had no need for information, knowledge or discussion.

All the children knew and understood that Lust was deadly and disordered and that fornication was a grave sin, a corruption and a scandal (but they weren't quite sure what fornication actually was).

So that's OK then. No need for condoms (horror) or sex education (avert your eyes and block your ears).

Surely their parents had never done It. They were all virgin births. Blessed.

SO THERE SHE WAS, Rapunzel, gifted with housework and mothering before she had even started her periods. Learning how to cook a roast, how to get whites whiter than white and best of all, how to please people. How to become the person that you have to be to get other people to like you, how to adapt and change into the woman that other people want you to be, how to lose yourself to the opinion of others, how to put them first and to put yourself away in a box and forget about it. Suffering herself in order not to upset others, doing anything, being anything to keep everyone happy. Exhausting, and, she would later learn, co-dependent.

Co-dependence: the art and addiction of sacrificing yourself to please others; martyrdom. Saintly. Such a good girl.

So, as she adapted, people pleased, whisked, polished and chivvied, she wiped her brow and tucked her burnished, auburn hair away behind her ears. First, she bunched it, then scrunched it, then plaited it, but still her hair grew and grew, looping into hoops caught at the base of her ivory neck.

As her womanhood bloomed, her porcelain skin shone virginal and when her mother said; "Rapunzel, Rapunzel let down your hair," they were astonished to see the wave of Titian silk spreading down her back, absorbing the candles lit at mass, exuding frankincense and myrrh.

Her hair was beautiful. A gift from God. So, there was no sin in celebrating His might by using it to advertise shampoo. Nothing naked, nothing smutty, nothing cheap, just back shots of her hair, undulating and glowing with health and vital vibrancy. Angelic.

Her mother was so proud; one daughter a model, one son a lawyer. The children had all turned out well. All but Rapunzel would marry good Catholic boys and girls when the time came. It was just a shame the other son had declined the priesthood; the ultimate accolade to parental virtue.

On billboards, in magazines, on TV, Rapunzel let down her hair and let it flow and shimmer her way into false self-esteem and enough money to buy her own place. Her beauty hid her frailty. The simpering of her agents and admirers plastered over her lack of self-worth. Her success was hollow, a scared, lacking-in-love-and-attention child hidden inside.

NTIL, ONE DAY her prince came to rescue her from the claws of commercialism and Catholicism. Swarthy and exotic, a man from a foreign land. Such a catch, such a sign of how desirable she was; to have such a handsome and powerful man interested in her was surely proof to herself and the world that she was, after all, worth something. 'Look what I can get' she thought, it was a big deal to enchant a prince from another land. He was so charming; Prince Charming; so seductive, so alluring, so, well, manly, and strong, and brooding; how could she resist?

Her parents were horrified, "He's a communist and he doesn't believe in God," her mother wailed, biting her tongue to stop herself from adding; "and he's a foreigner." They had raised Rapunzel to marry a good Catholic, Emerald man and in turn raise a huge Catholic brood; they were distraught and bereft.

Slightly smug, Rapunzel shrugged her lily-white shoulders, shook her scarlet hair and laughed at their parochial, narrow-minded ways before heading off into the sunset with her Prince Charming who showed her his huge, long, strong, erect tower and told her to make herself at home. He was so interesting, had such a good job. All the women loved him (she would only find out later just how much) and all the men wanted to be his friend.

He was a man of influence and stature. Of course she married him, for to have such amazing sex out of wedlock was a sin, she knew. They wined and dined and she listened to him regale his captured audience with all his tales. His stature was so huge that in his shade she withered away, getting smaller and smaller, finding it harder and harder to leave their ebony tower. He would dominate their dinner parties and she would hardly speak. People envied how happily married she was, lucky girl to be loved so.

But little did they know how, when the dregs were tipped and the crumbs wiped onto the floor (for her to sweep up later), he would, just for fun, use her like his own private punch-bag, a personal hobby. One, two, jab, stomach. One, two, jab, heart. One, two, jab, head. Horrific. But he couldn't help it, didn't mean it, he just got so jealous about her modelling. For a while the bruises didn't show in the places that the camera saw, and thank God she had all that hair to hide her shame and his finger marks.

It was clear it had to stop.

So, we'll skip through the years of ducking and diving, hiding and crying to find Rapunzel, now a mother, locked into her tower with a son and a daughter, waiting and wondering how to escape.

Not a good start to life for her little boy and girl. Rupunzel waited and wondered what to do. No new prince came to rescue her while Charming was off shagging other women. She was up high in her castle in the sky, sad, scared and all alone.

One day, hopelessly tearing at her hair in despair, she found that with it pulled from her face she could see clearly. Saw that her feet were way too high off the ground and her head too far in the clouds. Saw she was all alone. Saw it was down to her. Saw it was time to go

She plaited her long, red hair, flung it far from the window and watched as her children slithered safely down the tower to the safe woods below. "Come on mammy, now you, now you" came their calls and she saw that the only way out for her was to cut off her plait, to tie it to the rusting, blackened, iron bedframe and lower herself out to safety.

Which she did. Bravely hacking through the tendrils of approval, the tangles of other people's desires, until her head was shorn. She felt free without her hair, free and light; nobody could pull it this way or that.

She flew down her plait, giggling as she whizzed to escape and safety. She gathered her children from the woods where they danced a sprightly jig before heading to the solicitor's office.

While this may sound easy, do not be fooled. Our Rapunzel knew how to put on a brave face, she'd had a lot of practice. She had a secret hideaway; a house from her life before. But it was a struggle. Shorter hair was not so sexy, not so desired, not so provocative.

She eked money from modelling, film-extra-ing, working in a prison and a theatre company, (she could have been a great actress if her life had been different). Each day was heavy with working and mothering, alone. Making ends meet. Scrimping and scraping. Poor, and with no life of her own. This had not been the plan. 'Who wrote this script and where is my happy ever after?' she thought.

BUT RAPUNZEL SOON MET another prince. She was sure that this time she had chosen well; found Mr Right.

He didn't smoke, or drink, and she was so proud of how he had overcome his addictions to get to this clean-living place. He loved her shiny, shorter, more economical hair. So neat, so clean, so precisely cut; he hated mess and excess. He was charming and said all the right things. He wasn't foreign. Or a communist. A much better fit.

He spoke about his anger and his pain. Women really connected with him, really enjoyed the intimate ability he had to bear his soul and let them in. And he drew them in. He was manly too – soft but strong, rough but smooth. Idealised. Dreamy.

People loved him. Men and women. He belonged to a fellowship of men, strong men, doing men's work, reclaiming their masculinity, bonding. How cool is that? So intuitive and self-aware. How could she resist?

She couldn't and fell pregnant straight away. The fall of Eve. A fall into sin. An already divorced-unmarried mother-to-be, better get married soon to erase the shame.

Her daughter moved in with Prince Charming One, her father, and Rapunzel and her son moved in with Charming Two; his tower pristine and perfect and modern and white. The modern 'blended' family, mixing it all up; all mixed up.

No longer alone, a home and a happy family at last. This time she had got it right.

When the new baby was born, Charming Two strapped his new son to his manly breast and peacocked up and down the highways and byways parading and crowing:

"Look what a marvellous father I am. See how strong and sensitive I am caring for my newborn son. See how in touch with my feminine side I am to have the baby strapped to my breast. How I can be the provider and the protector and nurture too. Look at me, look at me. I am so wonderful, admire me, worship me, adore me."

Renaissance man reborn, again.

How inconsiderate of the baby to start wailing and screeching as babies do when they are hungry, tired or cold. How irritating that the noise was so loud and persistent; why was there no volume control? How could he meet his adoring crowds with such an unappreciative child in tow? How would that look? Charming Two had to retire from public life and all his fans (only temporarily, thank God).

How unfortunate that he seemed to have such an ungrateful wife, too; meeting him at the door, hysterical with accusations, her greasy, thinning, hair in plastic clips, berating him for the purple, squalling son and her milk-soaked T-shirt, dripping. What a mess she looked, all snot and tears and swollen udders and hair falling out, blocking the drains. Of course it was her job to clean them, all women have stitches after birth (he'd heard), she'd just have to get on with it. How ridiculous she was to worry about her son when he was with his father. What a hormonal mess. Yuk.

He should have known what a miserly, moaning, drag she was when she complained about their wedding. I mean, what kind of woman complains about an enormous wedding, over 250 strong, full of important men and women, useful contacts, powerful people and his acquaintances, his neighbours, his admirers. He even had space to invite a few of her friends and family and all she could do was complain about how she didn't know most of the guests. As if that matters; it was an occasion that would be talked about for years to come, it was so impressive.

So ungrateful.

When he had posted a beautiful photo of her on Facebook (an old photo from her modelling days, before she turned into a leaking, balding, scold), showing the world what a stunning wife he had acquired, she had made such a fuss. Why shouldn't he post pictures of his wife, showing the world how gorgeous she was, impressing his friends, making his followers jealous. He had married her, she was his. His limp and lame wife cried so much that in the end, a friend convinced him to take it down, but by the time he did, everyone had seen it. He made sure of that.

She was so demanding too, Rap, as he now referred to her. She wanted to defile his pristine stairway with a baby gate. She wanted ridiculous teddies for the baby. She wanted him to treat her now-teenage son the same way as his own daughter, as if that were fair? Why should he buy another man's son new clothes when the charity shop would do? His own daughter, of course, deserved the best. Of course, her son could carry his own (very heavy and old) TV upstairs, he was only crying because she had spoiled him, turned him soft. Of course her son could walk home from the same train station he had just picked his daughter up from; she was his princess, his little girl, she couldn't walk home alone. A big lumbering idiot like him? It would do him good! So he drove straight past and let the driving rain and searing wind toughen him up.

Nor did Rap have any understanding of his business. The stupid woman complained and cried when he told her that her older son could not have friends around to play, could not practice his piano, could not play his cello. How could he run a business from home with all of that racket, didn't they understand it was his house, his business, his money and he needed it just the way he liked it?

Then there was that time when Rap's sister (God knows which one, there are hundreds and each as dull as the other) came for dinner (burnt as usual, poor Charming Two had married a dreadful cook). Of course he was within his rights, as her husband, to scream and ball at her over dinner in front of her sister and brother-in-law. She was the one smoking all the time, swallowing down all her feelings, so unreconstructed, not like him, the modern man; expressive, cathartic, in touch.

Luckily Rap didn't have any friends to distract her from doing her household chores, keeping it all as shiny and polished as he liked it. She looked such a mess as she swept and polished and waxed, that no one would have wanted to be friends with her at all. She was always so tired, she'd never done a hard day's work in her life, didn't know she was born, she should try running a business.

And she was so clumsy, breaking cups and saucers, for which of course she had to apologise and pay. What was she thinking? Of course she couldn't simply use his coat, his sunglasses, his house, without his permission. She needed to learn boundaries. What was his was his. What was hers was his. How hard was that to comprehend?

One day she dared to suggest that he, her prince, might have ADHD. Big mistake. No more housekeeping money. A ban on the TV and radio, for it seemed to be filling her head with nonsense she was too stupid to understand.

BUT OF COURSE she was not stupid. This woman had escaped from a tower, had been brave enough to cut off her hair. That beautiful hair. And slowly but surely she started to regrow it. She needed to reclaim the narrative of her life. She saw her getting-bigger son standing up to her not-so-charming-after-all husband and her resolve grew; so did her courage.

This time she used the stairs, so much simpler. She borrowed money and moved out. She found a tower of her own and claimed it. She locked the door behind her and learned to be her own hero.

She taught her son to be kind and always nice to girls. She gave her daughter a room of her own and encouraged independence.

She learned how to change plugs and pay her own way.

She found she liked herself, with all her flaws and was surprised to discover that her confidence had not been hidden in her hair after all.

Who or what did she have to thank for her new life?

The fairy god mother?

No.

A priest?

No.

God?

No.

Her family and friends?

No.

Herself?

Yes. Herself.

Rapunzel rewrote her own story, in her own words, with her own hand, with her own thoughts. And she rose.

She rose, and rose and rose out of the dust, until at last she was standing, straight, sassy, haughty, sexy, rooted in the earth and reaching to the stars, grounded in her own wisdom.

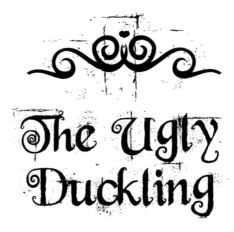

The Ugly Duckling

ONCE UPON A TIME there was a family of ducks. There was a daddy duck and a mummy duck and two sister ducks who happened to be twins. They lived together in a very normal corner of a very ordinary pond. All the ducks on the pond looked the same. They washed their beaks on Sunday and kept their nests tidy and their wing feathers oiled.

Daddy duck was very quiet and hardly made a squeak, let alone a quack. He liked to hide away, quietly watching dragonflies hover and the frogspawn pop, then splot, then wiggle, then hop in the hazy, spring sun.

Mummy duck was very bossy. Spit, spot, she liked the nest to be cleaned daily, fish to be eaten daintily, ablutions to be completed privately and for ducklings to do exactly as they were told. She ruled the roost. Her morning quack-call brought the sisterlings to attention, tummies in, beaks straight, wings neatly folded, feet webbed; attention!

The first duck-twin-ling was a good girl. She did what she was told, was neither good, nor bad, elegant nor clumsy, loud nor quiet. In fact, she was not very interesting at all.

The slightly younger duck-twin-ling was a different kettle of fish. Young duck-twin-ling was bright. Her glazed feathers reflected the sun's morning rays with just a little more sparkle than the other ducks'. Her sharp eyes could spot a fish in the murky depths (her mother had complained to the duck-council about the state of it), her quick beak could snaffle down a snack in a tail flick – "Watch your weight, daughter of mine." She could sense when the wind was turning, when the fog was rising and when the kids from the local village were coming with their mouldy, soon-sodden loaves.

It really irritated the other ducks.

To make matters worse, young duck-twin-ling was whitey-grey. But ducks on this pond, this small, fenced, pond, were brown and green. I ask you!

Young duck-twin-ling was inquisitive too:

"Mummy? What is that big green duck doing to the smaller brown duck? Why is it on the brown duck's back?"

"Don't look darling."

"But why is it grabbing the brown duck's neck? Mummy? Why is the brown duck drowning?"

"That's just what ducks do darling."

"But the brown duck doesn't like it. She is trying to get away."

"It's perfectly normal and acceptable darling. That is how mummies and daddies fall in love and make babies."

"Oh."

Occasionally, just occasionally, some of the white ducks from the Big Smoke would land for a family picnic on bank holidays, causing consternation and complaining for the local duckulation, but even they had yellow beaks and were low, slung, plump, tasty-looking beasts, nothing like young duck-twin-ling.

Young duck-twin-ling often found herself alone. The other ducklings wouldn't play with her, they said she let the team down during hide-in-reed-seek; she was too easy to see; useless. So she got used to being alone. She was not unhappy and really quite enjoyed her solitary vigil of the mayflies bouncing in the short-lived summer air and the froglets, hip-hop-splashing across the slimy stones. She was happy enough.

NTIL SHE STARTED paddling-school.

It became clear that she didn't fit in anywhere. She didn't fit in with the Badlings – the hard ones you didn't mess with.

She certainly didn't fit in with the Braces – the fit, look-how-strong-we-are ones. She didn't fit in with the Flushes – the pretty look-at-my-azure-shimmer ones. And she didn't fit in with the Strings – the drum-and-bass-groove ducklings.

No, she did not fit in at all.

So, when the new goose started, for this was a comprehensive, multi-cultural, mixed-sex (but none of that LGBT stuff yet) school, she couldn't help but notice him.

He was a skein-head and could really shake his tail feathers. He could get down and groove with the Strings, he would flirt with the Flushes, he would work out with the Braces and he ruffled feathers with the Badlings; he was just so cool.

One day there was a Paddling-School trip down to the local river. They had to walk in pairs; one hen, one drake, or they couldn't go. They had been briefed – side by side, tight pairs, walk to the left, look out for oncoming cars, for oncoming cats and oncoming dogs as they waddled their way to the wider water. No quacking, no honking, no hissing; nothing to draw attention to themselves. Any duck or goose found fouling on the pavement would be taken back in disgrace.

Young duck-twin-ling longed to see the river. She had heard stories of its wide banks, its endless length, its swish-swashing current; like a slide, like a sledge, slip-sliding you away. Such larks. She had begged her parents to take her but they always had their wings full with the next brood. She really didn't want to miss the trip but she had no partner.

First duck-twin-ling noticed her sister's sadness and looked around for a match, finding only Skein alone, standing fluffing and preening in the centre of the paddling school. Nervously first duck-twin-ling approached him and pointed towards her sister. At first Skein laughed and shook his head, wiping his beak on his feathers to show his disdain at such a suggestion. But when she pointed again, urging him to turn, he looked around, shrugged, and scuffed his feet as he swaggered his way towards the young duckling. He motioned, with a nod of the head, that she should fall in step, slightly behind him.

SHE DID.

Young duck-twin-ling was flattered and confused. His strutting and honking and beady eyes frightened her but there was something magnificent about having one so strong and fierce pay such attention to grey-white, unremarkable fluff like hers.

Once at the river, he left her to do more exciting things with more colourful fowl, but grudgingly deigned to walk home with her, one step ahead. He liked to be one step ahead. Older and larger, he always made sure he made it clear to her that she must walk behind.

So it continued. They would bump into each other in the play pond, she would edge up beside him in diving lessons, he would tease her in wing maintenance classes, and she would trail after him during take-off and landing classes. Truth be told, though he would never admit it, she was rather good at all her lessons. In fact, she was one of the brightest, most talented ducks on the pond, but he didn't want to let her know that, who wants a duck girlfriend who's going to show you up? He was the drake, he was a skein-head, she had to know her place.

He would laugh at her bookish knowledge of pond flora and fauna, of her understanding of water currents and the effect of global warming on the pond's microclimate. He would mock her for her quick calculations of the ever-expanding newt population and her scientific knowledge of the effect of pond algae on oxygen levels. Her knowledge of duck languages was encyclopaedic and she won prizes for her projects on The Role of Ducks in the Second World War, The Effect of Changing Air Currents on Duck Migration and Duck Crime and Deviance. In the Paddling School year book, she was deemed the 'Duck Most Likely To Go Far'.

And he hated it.

He hated it all.

She was such a swot. He honestly didn't know why he put up with her. He had to show her who was boss. So, when Skein was hanging with the Strings he would laugh at her lack of tone and rhythm. He could play the guitar with such ease, such panache and she was so gauche and clunky, practising her chords over and over whilst he was just a natural.

When he flirted with the Flushes, he made sure she knew how unsexy she was, how plain, how dull, how big, how white, how unsatisfactory.

When he worked out with the Braces he would flex his muscles, puff up his chest and wipe the sweat off his sleek, enamelled feathers and laugh at her pathetic, weak, wing stretches.

When he ruffled feathers with the Badlings, he would sneer at her goody-two-webbed-feet and leave her behind. He was just so cool. The Flushes would coo and quack and simper over his pectorals and the drakes all wanted to be like him. He was never alone, he was the leader of the raft, of the brace, of the flock.

He was everything that she was not. He was social, she was shy. He had loads of friends, she had few. He was confident, she was insecure. He knew he was perfect, she could only see her flaws. He was gorgeous, she was too big, too white, too awkward. He was funny and witty and quick, she was thoughtful, reflective and quiet. You could hear his quack from one end of the pond to another, she barely made a hiss. He liked to party and groove, she liked nothing more than a cup of pond soup and a good book.

She really was so lucky to be with him, she was punching up (he told her), she should be grateful he even let her smooth his feathers when they ruffled.

Her parents hated him. He was never welcome in her corner of the pond and her mother made it clear that she could do better. But the getting-older twinling felt rebellious, felt grown-up, felt so womanly and hen-like standing by her poor, misunderstood duckman. They couldn't tell her what to do; she wasn't a duckling anymore and she would show them, she would splash around with anyone she liked. So there. Try and stop me.

They couldn't, much as they would have liked to.

They wanted her to go to one of the best universities; she could have flown the nest to either Oxford or Cambridge Ponds, or maybe even their streams, possibly even their fastest stretches of river, she was bright enough. She could have been gliding around their historic spires and pecking on their immaculate cloisters, but she didn't even apply. She wanted to stay with Skein and Skein had only got offers from inner city watering holes, canals and ditches – Shore-ditch, Red-Ditch, Droit-ditch, you know the kind of places. Urban, redbrick sink holes with emptied cans of lager floating above rusting, drowned prams and supermarket trolleys in the fag-butt-dregs.

SO SHE FOLLOWED HIM to the Swamp and struggled to keep her head above the rising tide of his jibes and threats and taunts. She wasn't cool enough for his crowd and what on earth would one so sleek and toned as he want to hang around with her geeky crowd for? Her geeks didn't like him, saw how she had to waddle behind him, saw how he would pick and peck at her whitening plumes, heard how loudly he hooted whenever she waddled over to him, mocking her big black feet. He was now so much smaller in comparison, but Twinling just slouched and slumped and made herself smaller so he could feel as puffed up and plumped as his ego required. The geeks hated to see her treated that way.

Twinling learned to tiptoe, to soft-shoe-shuffle so as not to ruffle or incite him. Sometimes, when they were alone, trapped in an eddy or a backwash, he would rap, tap, jab, poke, hit or peck her. She knew he didn't mean to, he just got so frustrated, so angry with her; if only she was different.

One smoky-gnatted-night, when they were trapped in the eddies of a drain, he jumped on her.

"Mummy! What's that big green duck doing to the bigger white duck? Why is it on the white duck's back?"

"Don't look darling."

"Mummy, why is it grabbing the white duck's neck? Mummy, why is the white duck drowning?"

"That's just what ducks do darling"

"Why mummy? The white duck doesn't like it; it keeps trying to get away"

"It's perfectly normal and acceptable darling; that's how mummy ducks and daddy ducks make babies."

"Oh."

He was jealous about something, she couldn't remember what. He wasn't trying to kill her, honestly, he wasn't. He was just letting out his anger poor duck, letting out his testosterone-fuelled-wrath. He had only wanted her to listen, to see things from his point of view, to get her attention, goddamn her pesky-feathered-swots for hearing her croaking-hoarse-scared calls and coming to her rescue. Interfering nosy parkers.

But time moved on, the rows came, went and came back louder. She got used to the nipping and the pecking and the feel of his beak around her long, white neck. Even though he was smaller than her now, he had such power, such strength, such presence that she could never seem to shake him off.

Graduating Shore-middle-droit-ditch, they moved back to the pond but he was way too big for such small fry now and she didn't like her parents and the local duckulation seeing her bruises and her tufts of missing down so it wasn't long before they flew the nest to build their own in another pond, even though they had nothing in common. She knew no different, she had been a mere duckling when they met, so even though she was now fully grown, a huge, black-footed, long-beaked, snow-plumed, Eiger of a duck, she couldn't see beyond her beak to ask herself if she deserved more.

Life carried on.

She joined the city-commute to be one of the first female ducks in software design, in spite of his jibes and honks that she couldn't do it, that she would never amount to anything. Yet she did amount to quite a lot; in cash and reputation. She flew the heights of respect within her industry where she felt like she belonged; working with other geeks who only quacked when necessary, and did so quietly. She felt competent and successful and yet not fulfilled – her hidden heart pined for the gleaming towers, the whispering-quads, the Ashmolean, the Isis or the Backs, the Ely and the Cam.

What of Skein? What did he do while she worked with screens from dawn to dusk, through blackbird, nightingale, owl call and sometimes lark? She wasn't sure but the poor drake, who earned double her monthly seed, couldn't afford to take her out or pay more than half of everything they could need. It made her poor and made him rich, but her good-quiet-father duck had always told her to stand on her own two webbed feet and pay her way, find her own worms and fish and algae and on a good day, a frog, and she could. So she did and didn't think twice about the seed he hoarded and ate alone or all the flights he took without her. She didn't resent his much-needed weekend fix of football, flying high over stadia and shitting on the opponents' balding, flabby heads; what larks! She would just have to work harder.

It is just as well she did, as she had no friends, no social life, no fun; work kept her sane and busy and fluffed. Over the years with Skein her geek-quack mates had drifted on different eddies, different currents and streams, anything to avoid him, and therefore her. At first they had tried to pull her along with them by her tail feathers, but she had resisted, loyally, and so could only stand alone in the shallows and watch them drift away.

So WHEN THE invitation to a wedding came, she blinked her beady yellow eye and looked again. But there it was, he and she invited on stiff white card, with golden undulating borders, smelling of opulence and caviar; yum.

The day came and they prinked and preened and fluffed and sleeked, but no matter how she did her feathers he found fault; too fluffy, too flat, too white, too fat. Her feet too wide, too black, her eyes too greeny-gold, like rotten pond weed. Waddling behind him, head bowed, neck curved earth-ward, they made their way into the splendidly clean bower of a south-city pond, all coy carp and plastic herons.

It was so good to see her child-duckling friends again, so lovely to be with ducks who liked her. When they suggested that she and Skein would be the next to wed, he scoffed and scorned that one as Peter Pan-ish and charming as he would never be tied down by one so clumsy and huge and white. He was too much of a catch, too fine, too free for such an ungainly, inelegant, unattractive shackling. 'I don't want to be with him', thought Twinling and watched him as he wandered off to have a fine time flirting, primping and grooming with the exotic mandarins, resplendent in their designer purple plumes with precise piping and flutes of ochre and gold.

So, for a while, she forgot about Skein, who forgot about her, and she started to enjoy herself. She chattered, hooted and trilled, she even giggled and gaggled and wiggled. She enjoyed herself until the heavy church clock struck twelve and she turned from a happy-clacky-plucky duck into one scared to go home with Skein. She had forgotten him totally for those golden hours and now felt his brooding, slouching, seething presence approaching. As they waddled home, alone, him staggering after drinking too much frog spawn and smoking too much pond weed, her heart sank.

He bullied her and prodded her and poked her and pecked his anger out; how dare she forget about him, laugh without him, talk without him, breathe without him, even if he was off laughing and talking and breathing without her? Didn't she know who was boss, didn't she realise how everyone was laughing at her really? Didn't she see how ridiculous she looked chattering and trilling and gaggling? Pathetic. Peck. Peck. Peck. Until her neck was bruised, her feathers were missing and her pillowy down scattered the dark, shards of stone over which they waddled.

Her fault. She only had herself to blame. She had brought it on herself.

She shut out her friends and worked harder. Her snowy white head bowed and her elegant neck stooped and kinked with age and screens and fear. Dawn to dusk, sunrise to sunset, lark to owl, work, eat, home to the barren nest where he would huff and fluff and peck and splash and then largely ignore her.

A mere greyish duckling when they had first met, and now, many years later, a mature pond dweller of 29, she had coaxed and cajoled him into a much longed-for break. They flew off to a warmer clime where the sun painted her snowy feathers pink and orange and the water, though salty, was warm and clear. She hadn't seen her reflection for so long in the murky half-light of dawn or dusk pond that when she looked down she was surprised to see a rather elegant undulating neck, a handsome ebony beak and two clear, yellow-gold eyes looking back at her. She liked what she saw and stretched out her wings in the sun, her strong wings, her powerful, extensive wings, her magnificent canopy of white, shimmering against the summer, blue sea. No longer the ugly duckling he had told her she was, she caught a glimpse of the Hermes, Iris, Eros she might allow herself to be. And she knew she wanted to be free.

She found the key to her escape along the esplanade, pecking at snail, frogs' legs, moules and frites. Lost in her daydreams, in a Skein-free world, on the eve of her 30th birthday. She didn't hear him calling. She didn't hear him quacking and squawking at her to heel and pay heed to him. She didn't hear the pounding of his wings and the flapping of his feet until he pounced on her, rubbing her snowy-white down into the sandy, warm clay beneath her heaving breast. He pecked and pecked and pinched and squeezed and bit and screeched. He bent her wing tips backwards to sprain against her back, he twisted her long, sinewy neck to glare in her closed eyes, he pulled and plucked at her underbelly until the down flew like thistle-froth into the forget-me-not blue yonder.

"Maman? Maman! What's that big green duck doing to the bigger white duck? Maman? Why is it on the white duck's back?"

"Don't look cheri."

"But the white duck is struggling Maman"

"That's just what ducks do mon cher."

"Pour quoi Maman? The white duck doesn't like it; it keeps trying to get away."

"You're right mon fils, it's not an acceptable way for the le pere to treat la mere; ce n'est pas how we treat people we love."

"Let's chase him away Maman!"

And so they did.

And so did Twinling.

SHE MOVED IN with her sisterling and didn't answer his calls, his honks or his screeches. Twinling's mother, sister, father and friends all cheered and were relieved to have her back in the home-pond safe and sound.

It wasn't easy, to start again. Skein didn't like Twinling, but he wouldn't let her go. He would turn up at sisterling's nest insisting on seeing Twinling. He told her she was mad and made her see a hypnotherapist. He told her he loved her so they went to Relate. He was best friends with sisterling's husband, which was a bit tricky all round, but even their shared drakery was not enough to insert himself back into Twinling's life. Twinling held onto her work, saw a solicitor and reclaimed her nest egg from under his rough, brown butt.

Twinling stretched her wings, eased out the stressed kinks in her serpentine neck and drew herself up to her full height; resplendent in her auric-halo of celestial white.

"You're a swan, a magnificent, majestic swan," swooned a Canadian goose at work. He was solid: anti-Fascist, environmentally sound, straight as a reed, reliable as algae, as transparent as the mirror-like sea. Someone she could trust.

This was not the faint fluttering of youth; the romantic whims of unrequited-rough-rejection and flirtation. Canada was a grown goose, a goose who had seen the world, a goose who could navigate the air currents and turbulence of the long flights of life. He could find his own food, he had his own friends, stood on his own, splayed, webbed feet.

She couldn't quite see the beauty in her that he saw, feeling still the pecks and nips of ugly-grey-oversized-ducklinghood, but they fell in love. Her parents adored him and welcomed him into their pond, their nest, their hearts. Canada showed her a different life, taught her how to belong, chased away her loneliness.

They had one gosling, then a cygnet and lived happily and ordinarily, sharing and caring, in a way she had never dreamed possible. As the children grew and stretched their wings, Twinling ventured forth with them to study once more; not in the turrets and currents of her dreams, but on a course which filled her heart and expanded her mind and showed her she wasn't too old or too slow or stupid.

Challenged, she started to look again at her reflection in the home-pond-pools. She started to see that she was not too big, or fat, or awkward. That she was not too white, too blank, too plain. That her neck was not too long, too snake like, too twisty. That her wings were not too wide, too pointy, too pokey, too hard.

She slowly began to see that she was a swan.

She couldn't quite believe it. She rippled the shallows and waited for them to settle before looking again, but still she saw, ankle deep in green water, a swan.

She was a swan.

A swan!

Can you imagine?

As she let the waters settle and her reflection still, she allowed herself to look closer and began to see other things, too. She was not too quiet or geeky or shy. She was not tuneless, talentless or thick. She was not an embarrassment, a laughing stock or an ungainly klutz.

She even tentatively allowed herself to believe that Canada found her sexy, attractive, funny, loyal and kind. That her friends liked her warm wit, her listening ear, her patient, welcoming wings. That her children

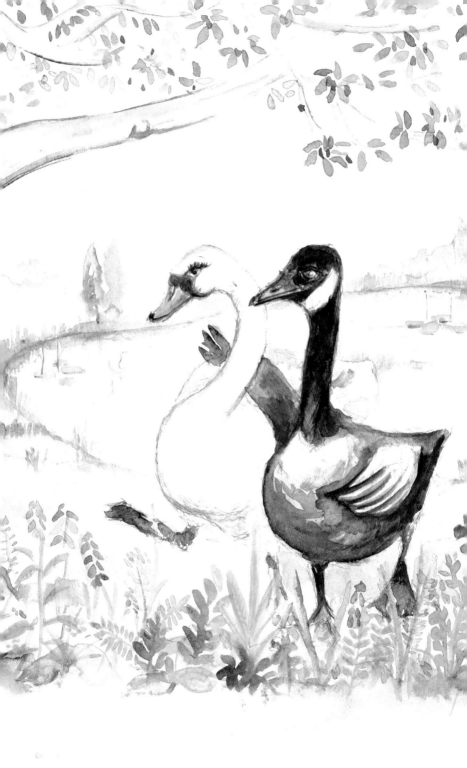

thought she was the best mother this side of the moon. She found her brace, her raft, her team, her flock and found that she fitted right in.

As the seasons turned, the frost thawed from the banks and the wind whispered of warmth and light, she started to shake off the dust of self-loathing. She shook the drops of fear from her winter down. She groomed the self-criticism out of her wings and tail. She smoothed away her anxiety and accepted the love her family gave her. As the snowdrops poked their swan-like heads above the iron soil, she allowed herself to borrow and believe in their hope, in their ability to reinvent themselves, growing bigger and stronger year after year.

Sometimes waves of anger, resentment and regret from the Skein-past would threaten to swamp her, but Canada was always there to help her to stiller waters. A simple goose, he didn't really understand her skein-life-scars, but swam beside her, quietly, through her storms.

Her mother and father passed from their nest to the great-sky-beyond and her gosling and cygnet flew the nest full grown. Sisterling remained her right-wing-woman and her friends loyally and lovingly circled her life.

On summer evenings you might see a goose and a swan companionably waddling slowly around a pond, taking their time to smell the buttercups, laugh at the dragonfly-trapeze, pass the time with the ducks and to chortle at the antics of the duck-goslings and cygnets as they play hide and seek in the rushes and reeds.

Such small things are where happiness lies.

"Mummy! Look at that black and white goose walking with the big, white swan. Where are they going Mummy?"

"For an evening stroll round the pond darling."

"Why are they together Mummy?"

"Because they like each other darling."

"But they're not the same."

"That doesn't matter darling, as long as they are happy."

"Why are they pecking at the grass Mummy?"

"Because that's what swans and geese do."

"They look happy Mummy."

"Yes darling, they do."

Beauty and the Beast

ONCE UPON A TIME there was another Beauty.

I know, I know, isn't it dull how women are defined by their looks rather than their brains, and this lot are bright women, not your typical victims of abuse – because there are no 'typical' victims of abuse. So, let's call this woman Jane, and no she wasn't plain; in fact her looks shouldn't matter at all, but of course they do, as you will later see, as you read on.

So there once lived a girl called Jane, who was a good little girl. Her life was all polished shoes and ironed socks. She watched her Ps and Qs and could dot her Is and cross her Ts. She was very properly brought up.

Little girl Jane loved her daddy as many girls do. He worked away, on boats or down mines or even in an office, she was never quite sure but his coming and going would break her heart and that was all she knew.

I could tell you that when he came home he would jiggle Jane on his knee, that he would present her with fine, exotic gifts, that she was his golden girl, but Jane can't remember if he did. He just came and went and when the adult Jane saw a coat like his, a Crombie in a film, walking away from the camera, it made her cry.

And Jane had a mother, but she is a bit-part player, significant only in her lacking and absence so that's enough of her for now.

Childhood came and went, and Jane watched as the pixelated, black and white screen of her life came into sharper focus – in bloodied colour – when her period started and her breasts budded. Now more womanish, her father played a different note.

Sliding into the bathroom as she dressed, ignoring her shy shame and hasty coverings, his huge fingers would graze pubescent skin, pulling up barely-there bra straps and smoothing down unwanted slip-wrinkles over her filling-out thighs, ignoring her downcast-averted-confused blue eyes. She dare not send him away and had not the strength to lean against the lockless door to keep him out. Life hovered on the jamb, hesitant and confused, not knowing what to do.

Some days Jane's father would loom into the bathroom and take root on the side of the bath and stare with hot coals as she finished her ablutions, pointing out when she missed a bit, and insisting that she washed some part better than others, now that she was a woman. She would later think she caught him sniffing the air to catch her adolescent scents, she often wondered if she imagined seeing his mouth water. Terrified, her fumbling fingers couldn't ever close the clasps to safety or haul up her protective underwear fast enough to escape his lascivious looking.

Then there were the beatings. Finger marks on face-slaps, fist grabs around slender wrists, blue-blushes around her eyes where silly girl must once again have walked into a door. Why did no one notice? Or perhaps they did and were too scared to speak, she certainly was, never telling a soul. Life pulled its knees up tight into its chest at night and buried its bruised face into the tear-damp pillow, sobbing itself to sleep.

Jane's mother is only important for her lack and absence. She offered no protection, no safety, no help and no comfort other than "Shush, shush, shush he doesn't mean it."

But of course he did.

Slap, bang, thank you ma'am.

Jane came to hate him and planned her escape into the doors of the nearby college. She didn't do as well as she might have, nor would you if you had your father leering at you and beating you daily. Why did nobody notice? Perhaps they didn't dare, didn't care.

A tiny wee thing, nervously undernourished, she found her friends and a boyfriend too, who chastely held her hand and thought her beautiful. "You're not going out looking like that, looking like a prostitute!" her father boomed, shaking her pre-date nerves more firmly to her knees and sending her wet-behind-the-ears-nice-boy date scurrying. Ending that blossoming romance.

HEN ONE DAY she met her prince at last. He was incredible; a PE student, all muscles, masculinity, sinews and sweat. He chose her and his pheromones, his good looks and charm knocked her sideways and into his waiting arms. His name was Rodney. Life perked up, lighting its eyes, blooming its skin, daring to hope and imagine.

Now, Jane had been brought up a good Catholic girl, no sex before marriage and all that, but what nobody knows, no one can tell, and so before she succumbed to Rod's magnetism and spells she very sensibly whispered "We need to be careful. I ought to wait until I'm on the pill."

Rod glared, Rod snarled, and then Rod sprouted hairs from his nose and his ears (which she was sure were slightly longer than before). "Are you refusing me?" he snarled. "Nobody refuses me!" he slathered from his blackening lips and his elongated snout. She rubbed her eyes and could not believe her ears or eyes as she watched him launch himself at the door frame, flexing his pectorals, which were sprouting hairs, as he pulled himself, muscles bulging, upwards. "Nobody!" he growled, flashing fangs she'd not seen before and balling his giant hairy fist to punch it right through the door before pinning her to the bed and inserting himself into her erstwhile virginity until she was sore; too scared and weak against his mighty-bearing-down to even contemplate resistance.

He left her on the bed and prowled out, slamming the door.

Dazed and confused, she thought she must have been seeing things. This was not what she had dreamed off. This was the wrong fairy tale. He had huge eyes (all the better to see her with); a big hairy snout (all the better to smell her with); sharp teeth (all the better for biting her with); and long, curved claws (all the better for flaying her still-tender skin with). She must have made the whole thing up in the dark corners of her imagination. Best get some sleep. Things would be better in the morning. Life tried to soothe her broken sleep, holding her safe in its arms through the long, troubled mazes of dreams.

The next day, when Rod (normal features returned) pleasantly circled her waist in the dinner queue she leaned into him relieved that the nightmare was over. He was charming, he was fun, she was the envy of all the girls, what a catch she'd snared.

Snared.

The snare was his, not hers, but she didn't see it catch and tangle around her, tying her in, tying her up, tying her to him.

THE FIRST TIME he punched her in the face, blacking her eyes, she didn't see the transformation coming, just caught a glimpse of his blood-cursed eyes glaring at her angrily before gristle made contact with bone, shattering with a guttering crunch.

"Never speak to me like that. Never ever do that again" he snarled through curled lips. She had no idea what she had done and was so dizzy with pain, the only thing she saw was the grizzled grey of a bristled tail before it faded away through tear-drenched eyes.

Later, back at her parent's house, her father madly mocked, "Did you walk into a revolving door? Good for him because somebody needs to tame you."

Her heart shrunk into a tiny jewelled case and locked the door behind it.

"At least he's Catholic," said her weak and wavering mother. Jane threw away the key and watched as Hope took flight and dashed its head, trying to escape through the barred windows, before spiralling downwards to the cold, slabbed floor.

Things got worse, here a tripping foot (or paw – she never was sure), there a slap, daily humiliations and constant scarring to her still-young soul. Life trudged onward, covering the battered-bruising as best it could.

Rod was adventurous, exciting and wild so when he suggested they go travelling, she dreamed of holding hands in St Mark's Square, kissing under the Eiffel Tower, people-watching on the Spanish Steps. Her heart beat for the galleries they would admire, the fountains they would splash in, the parks that would shade them, the food they would feed each other. Picture-postcard scenes of bliss, which would never be hers to send.

The food was greasy road-side-fodder, the cafés and rooms cheap and filthy, the trains overcrowded and late. No hands were held, there was no tender caressing in the Boboli Gardens. Instead he walked ahead, walked away, ignored her pleas for help and patience as she dragged her heavy backpack through the dusty, blazing streets; her back aching and her eyes stinging. Alone.

When they were back on familiar soil and she had washed the dust from her hair, and scrubbed the dirt from under her nails, she finished with him. Life cheered and took her out to play with friends.

At first she was astonished and wryly amused by his howling, his sorrow. This wasn't what she had expected, his protestations of devastation, his knee-hugging-clinging entreaties to have him back, to heal him with her love, his threats to kill himself if he couldn't have her.

Extracting herself from his sticky supplications, she turned her back on him and joined the world of fun and friends, dancing and flirting, laughing and playing and being young and free.

She felt his presence before she saw him, felt her spine tingle as she giggled and wiggled to the dark throb of the DJ. "It's not over yet," he hissed. Her heart pumped faster, she wiped the new sweat from her palms and turned away again to follow her friends to the bar, to the kebab stall in town, to the taxi rank in the small hours before dawn. He tracked her, trailed her, shadowed her every step, her every gesture. He lurked in the corners, in the gutters, in the queues; glaring, brooding, hunched and ready to pounce.

Her friends didn't like him, wanted him gone, rolled their eyes, turned their backs, changed the subject, but his hooks were in her and she couldn't shake him off. He trailed her to work, stalked her home, pursued her in the supermarkets. He cajoled her as she walked, stroked her when she was still, charmed her with promises of love-tender-caring, of sweet-night-passion, of the-love-of-my-life, of I-can't-live-without-you. He flooded her, swamped her, groomed her, suffocated her with his saccharine promises, sweeping her closer to his arms.

And so, reader, she married him and in so doing plighted her troth, promised to obey and signed away her right to say "No". For now, in the law's eyes, he could insist, persist, push and penetrate without her permission, without her volition, under submission, for she was his; his property, his goods and chattels. Rape didn't exist inside the marriage bed; for consent was given once and for all at the alter and couldn't be altered thereafter at all.

What could she say? Who could she tell? Her friends had left, shaking their heads in disbelief at the church door. Her father had winked and nudged her betrothed to display the bloodied sheets of the wedding night and her mother had slipped by, as insubstantial as a dream; head down, shoulders bowed, shoes shuffling across the cold, stone floor.

So when they moved near to his mother, she had hoped for better there.

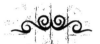

BUT SHE SHOULDN'T have counted her chickens for rotten apples ne'er fall far from cankered trees.

It was only later, much later, that Jane would hear how Rod's mother had dragged her wailing pre-school boy to the woodshed to teach him a lesson for some unknown infant crime. How she would leave him there through the smoking twilight into the ebony hours and into dawn. How his starved fingers would scrabble for old cat biscuits, lick water from the frost window panes to ease his thirst. How he quickly learned that his crying, his imploring, his hammering, his screams led to nothing. The old iron-coloured back door firmly locked against him and glimpsed only through the warped wood through which the wind accompanied his howling. Released on his mother's whim, battered again for being fetid with his own excrement, blackened with coal-saw-dust and grime, he would then cling to her with all his might, loving her harder that she might in turn love him.

He only later told Jane of his terror at the suffocating darkness and the serpentine tendrils of cobwebs washing his face with spider feet. Her heart broke to hear of the rats brushing past his small, bleeding hands, clutched in terror over his eyes, trembling from trying to tear his way free of the dank, rotting, rank, grave. Her heart became tender, she wanted to mend him, to heal him, to make him whole and safe and secure. She knew only too well what it was like to have a parent who scared you.

What no one but Life saw, what no one would have believed, as the

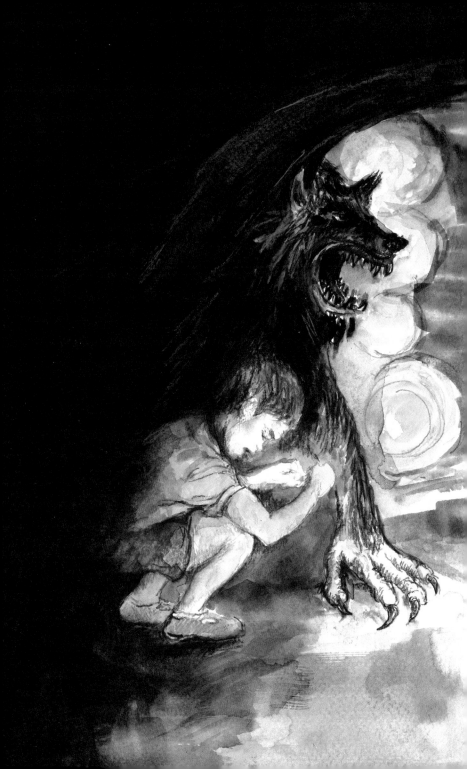

woodshed incarcerations increased in their frequency and duration, was that Rod started to change, to turn, to mutate through each lost and soulless hour. Coarse needles of bristles would pierce and rupture his fragile infant skin, his button nose would crack and split as a bony snout forced its way forward, sniffing, slavering, ready to devour that which tortured him. Canines sliced their way through dribbling gums, forcing the budding milk teeth out of their way. Yellowed scythes split and splintered the still soft nails, from bitten and snagged to daggers and knives. His backbone stretched, extending and pulling each soft vertebra until his coccyx shattered making way for a tail. Transformed, his red eyes dried of tears and tearing, his fur coat itching with mites and fleas, he would drop to his haunches, and howl, in full moon or none, howl for love where there was none.

He told Jane of the torture, but not of his shape-shifting. Who would have believed it had he told? All Jane imagined was a foetus-shaped bundle of rags on the woodshed floor when the door was opening in the cold grey of dawn. A bundle of rags who grew up to be a boy, then a man. Her man.

Jane's new friend Kate would, over cups of tea, recall school day whisperings of what the teachers thought made little Rodney so withdrawn, what made his too-young face crease with frowns. Kate warned how even then, there was something about him she didn't like, something menacing and cold, how sometimes in the changing rooms after Rhythm and Movement she was sure she'd glimpse a tufted tail disappearing below his schoolboy shorts. "No one liked his mum," she'd recall, "they said she had the evil eye and even crossing your fingers couldn't protect you from her curse."

It made Jane squirm to watch mother and son together now; his fawning, caressing, his adoration, his love. Their pawing, kissing and stroking made her feel sick.

She learned to ignore it, outside life was good. A good job, great colleagues, recognition and success; she was well liked and laughed a lot. Life looked almost happy. She could almost forget the growlings and pawings, the slaverings and the prowling when she focused on work. Her looking glass life, happy on one side, on the other a mere shadow, a reflection of how he wanted her to be.

LIFE BLUSHED and flushed to see how the husband dressed his barbie-doll, all strapped tight in fitted sheaths and tittering heels, barely able to hold her aloft as she teetered into work. Rod watched to see the heads she turned, a beauty, with blond hair, trussed up for office politics, the cut and thrust of the workplace. It made him feel so big, so hard, so strong to know that he had chosen what touched her skin, that he had licked her flesh raw with his desire, that he knew the mauvish reminders of their intimacy that lay laced beneath the dog-tooth checks and twin-set pearls. He liked a bit of cut and thrust himself.

At first she liked the dressing up, she liked that he cared enough to choose and fit, to match and pair. The sheer silk stockings and kinky underwear seemed signs of his desire, markers of his territory, the outlining of what was precious to him. She felt his desire press in on her as he watched him fuck her from behind in front of her blanching mirror, at first feeling the fairest of them all, then tarnishing as the leather lost its lustre and the rubber split. She began to hate it. The slime of his semen made her flesh retract and withdraw and her eyes searched ever-downwards avoiding the mirror on the wall, not liking what she saw or who she had become. Maybe this was marriage, maybe this was sex, maybe was this was love, she wasn't sure. How could she be when she'd only ever read about Happy Ever After.

THEN JANE FELL PREGNANT and from the first moment of bubbling life, she loved her curled-up-tucked-in-tight son. After son one, came son two; the mother years passing in a blur. They were a triangle of love, rarely disturbed by the predatory sire. Jane was grateful, for their triad was a magical realm of sticky fingers, tousled hair and carpet-play-kingdoms where The Right and The Good reigned peaceably. The babies saved Jane's skin for a while, protecting her from fists and kicks but could not cast a charm strong enough to sift out the verbal assaults, to protect or defend her mind from the words which wormed in and lodged there.

These were the years of bedtime stories, bubble baths and Lego. The three would adventure through pine-lit woods, scramble into rock pools and shriek with glee as they sausage-rolled down the hill to her loving arms below. She felt blessed by their opulent-corn-gold-hair, their chubby-petal toes, the way they would baby-suck her chin and her fingers, her nose and make her laugh until the tears would stream down her face to join with their shining, watching eyes. She loved the boys with the flesh from her bones and the air from her lungs; their laughter and antics, their clowning and parading were welcome rainbows in the stormy clouds. Sometimes their father would take them to play tennis or football and for those moments, she would re-kindle Hope and imagine that they really could be a family, that he really would be the husband and father of her dreams, ignoring the scowls and the taunts, the mocking and the hurts, the silent acquiescence to unwanted penetration so as not to wake the babies.

The lullaby years lulled her into a dream of nearly-happy living and she dared to hope that all would be well. And well enough it was until she outgrew the baby-grows and buggy and made her bright and hopeful way back to work.

Work where her make up didn't smudge with fear and where her hair bounced free of baby puke and soggy biscuit. Work where people laughed at her jokes, where she could share her views and disagree without the fear of fist or foot. Work where women wanted to be her friend and where some men saw her pale freckles and huge corn-flower eyes and felt their knees weaken and their fantasies expand. Work where she was free to think, free to excel, free to be.

He hated it. Believing he couldn't trust the slag he would control what she wore, he would watch from the window, marking time, checking minutely for signs of detours without his permission. He would follow her into the city, patrolling the pavements outside her office block, escorting her from the premises in virtual arm locks. And behind the respectable middle-class door the beating started again.

He would drag her up the stairs by the scruff of her collar and slam open the bedroom door. Grabbing her hair, he would yank back her head; forcing her to fall so he could drag her dazed and tiny body by its blond ponytail across the polished floor to slam her head into the wall "I'm sorry. I'm sorry," was all she could think to cry, not knowing what she was apologising for but feeling his ferocity and fearing for her life as the blows rained down with words of shame; "Tart, witch, bitch, cunt, whore," a never-ending assault on flesh and brain.

Then he would rape her. Wherever she was slumped, regardless of blood and bruising, regardless of the clumps of dismembered hair. "Please don't, please don't, please don't," she would sob, but he would flip her over to muffle her cries and shove himself harder and faster inside. Smashing her face into the floor, grinding her nose against the wood, polishing it with her blood. And when he'd cum, he'd finish her off with a good kicking to kidneys and spleen, to guts and groin, leaving her foetal and flayed.

A daily diet of slaps for dinner not served to order, punches for the radio on too loud, kicks for his ironing not done on time. She never knew who would be coming for tea, man or beast. There were days when Rod would arrive all good looks and charm, chatty-daddying tea-time eggy soldiers with their two young boys, only to revert to his wolverine ways over the washing up.

She told no one, hid the bruises which he considerately often made beneath her clothes. The school gate mums assumed she'd been over-zealous in her marital conjugations the night before on seeing how she hobbled bow-legged to wait for her home-time boys. The night before, when unable to find the remote control and finding that his coffee had gone cold, he had slammed her backwards into the sofa, winding her, whiplashing her neck, before pulling her knees apart and slamming his fist hard into her vagina. "Cunt." Fist crunching, bone. Only when he was sweaty and tired from his punchbag exertions, did he leave her alone.

And still she told no one. Until the day came when he sliced a plate into her head, washing her hair in blood. Calling Kate with sticky crimson fingers; "I need to go to the doctor," she said "I can't see to drive". "You have to tell someone," insisted Kate whilst driving and passing wads of folded toilet roll to stem the tide of crimson.

S O THE RHYTHM of their relating changed, cycling around harm caused, help sought, her brave and loyal brother summoned to the rescue only to stood down in the face the Rod's humble, begging apologies. Rod would fall to all fours and plead to be forgiven, insisting that he loved her, adored her but that she had driven him to it, whatever it was, it was always her fault, something she'd done was the cause. He had never meant to, didn't want to, couldn't help it, she had made him, if only she'd been different, been more loving, quieter, kinder, sexier, tidier, didn't she know how he loved her so? He would cling to her knees, bring her presents, stroke her hair, promise her the world, a brighter future, anything to show he cared.

And because she had children, because she was so exhausted, so confused and bemused, because the wounds had healed and the bruises faded, she let herself fall for his ruse and stay.

But she was young, and pretty and smart with a head full of dreams and a heart full of Hope even though she had locked it away. So when a young Spaniard walked into her office, all kindness and caring, all tender attention, she turned to Life and held out her hand for her heart, and opened the key, to open the lock to give her heart away to the dark-skinned-limpid-eyed beauty holding her hand.

Life didn't judge her for the stolen walks, the touching hearts, the whispered words over paperclips and files. Life knew how she had ached and pined since she was a child, for one man to love her, to love her and leave her whole, leave her intact, not molested like her father or the beast. Life saw how she needed to feel beautiful, how welcome this young man's laughing eyes were, how they smoothed her fearful brow. Life saw the young man hold her in horrified disbelief as she told her dark and twisted tales of home, saw him gasp and well up at the welts on her lily skin, the burned scabs of fags, the purple veins of bruising.

Their love-making was a tendrilling of feelings, tingling across their gossamer skin, releasing the two bodies into one sweet undulating pulsation, one deep inhalation, one long sigh of peace. She would cry to be held so deeply, so tenderly, so gently if only for a stolen hour. Their secret world was hidden from photocopiers, the traffic lights, the garden gate and the suspicious front door.

Only a neighbour noticed; "My! You do look well our Jane, anyone would think you were in love." If only she hadn't let the corner of her mouth rise, if she had kept the twinkle from her eye, if her shoulders had slouched, her gaze turned downward, then maybe the neighbour would never have teased the Beast about what he and his wife must have been up to, to made her shine so brightly.

F ONLY. THEN she might have avoided the bashed, smashed, cracked, bleeding revenge of her cuckolded spouse. If only. Then she might have seen her lover once before he was relocated for his own safety, a new office, a new marble floor. If only. Then she might have lived free of the straightjacket the Beast tied her in, releasing her only for chores and work and to be his whore.

Of course Rod went running to his mummy, telling tales of what the nasty lady had done to mummy's little boy. The hag swelled and swore and as swift as a knife cutting a vein, pushed into Jane as she stood, bruised, stooped, ironing.

"Bitch! Witch! I curse you witch! You have ruined my dear son's life and I will make you pay!" screeched the harridan, spitting fury across the washing pile, poking her poisoned finger into Jane's broken heart. "My son has done everything for you and you have betrayed him! I will make you suffer. I will make you wish you had never been born." The hurled words hurricaned across the laundry, and whipped at Jane's eyes, tearing them, scratching them, stinging them until she would stand no more.

Roaring, Jane launched herself, shielded by the melting iron; "I have so many times wished I had never been born! You have no idea what happens in this place!" Holding the heat towards his mother's face she gathered herself and told, through clenched jaws and tense gut, how her darling son had mutilated, suppurated, asphyxiated, micturated, punctured and starved her, how he had shamed her and blamed, her, how he had blocked the drains with handfuls of her hair and washed out her mouth with bleach. The forced penetrations, the rapes, the thousand intimate instances of humiliation and pain were too shameful to yell even in fury, even in validation and protection of herself.

"Get out of my house!" scorched Jane, and off flew the harpy to find her son and bring him home for Jane's reckoning. Jane phoned her brother terrified, her brother who, many times before had come to save her with his baseball bat and many times was met with charming Rod explaining away a confused and 'pre-menstrual' Jane. "You know how hysterical women can get at that time of the month don't you?"

"Come quickly. Come quietly. Come now." She stole upstairs to collect her hiding-behind-the-bedroom-door-with-their-fingers-in-their-ears boys. Heart pumping, fingers sliding around trembling locks, she clutched two trembling hands and guided them into her waiting, faithful car.

HER BROTHER was a marvel, keeping them safe and sound for days, but she had to get back to work, the children had to go to school, they couldn't live their lives hiding behind the tasteful drapes of calm and welcome suburbia. Hysterical gremlins ran riot in her mind; 'What if he takes the children from school? What if he doesn't bring them back? What if he harms them? Some men kill their own children. What if he takes them somewhere I can never find them again? Where will we live? How will I support us all?' Jane knew she couldn't stay with her brother, but she didn't know how she could leave, where she should go.

Head in hands of despair she didn't at first understand the commotion, didn't notice the winged flagration gathering momentum in the firmament. Life raised her sorry head and pointed out, with a wink, Jane's mother astride a crimson dragon, blazing a trail towards the Beast's house. The neighbours craned and crooked in amazement, nudged and whispered their thoughts and theories as to what the once timid mouse was doing straddling such a magnificent salamander between her strong and matriarchal thighs.

"No one harms my daughter and gets away with it! Not any more! Never again!" Came the virago's war cry, straightening her spine and pushing back her shoulders as she came into land on the postage-stamp-plot of suburban drudgery that Jane had called home.

She bestrode the garden path like a colossus. The moss hid in cracks, the flowers shuttered their petals, the worms, confused, tore themselves in half and went on to live a soil-safe double life far from the madding crowd. Spurs rattling, leather chaps shielding her thighs, she hammered Thor-like on the door.

Charming Rodney answered, inviting her in for cuppa and a chat. But this late-translated Circe unsheathed her mortal sword of truth and held it up for all to see, listing his crimes so all could hear. "Oo, this is better than any daytime TV," whispered the spineless gossipers who had heard Jane's cries and turned away. "She's mad," he shrugged, winking at his mates. But the wind was turning. "Tis true. Tis true," the whispers grew until, gathering as a wave they crashed through the door, gathering his flotsam and detritus and sweeping him.

AND SO IT CAME to pass that Jane reclaimed the family home while The Beast skulked off to his mother's lair to lick his wounds and silently seethe. Jane cleaned and scrubbed the floors where her blood had long since dried. She emptied her cupboards of the sex-clothes he had bought her. She wiped the mirror clean of his greasy fingerprints, but no matter how hard she polished, she couldn't erase the sights the mirror had seen. She helped her children start to unpack, not just their toys, but their tensions. Reading bedtime stories she would stroke their hair and their brows, trying to wipe the worry signs away. Life carried on, wobbling on unsteady legs, but moving forward step by step.

Their solicitor, naive to signs of abuse, suggested mediation or Relate, believing that he was dealing with a man not a Beast. Obediently Jane went, her solar plexus so tight that it hurt to breathe while he was inhaling the same air as her. The counsellor listened, non-judgemental but alert, saw Rod's vitriol leaking, his jaw tense. Saw Jane's lips turn blue as she iced with fear. The solicitor made the call, the courageous call which saved her; "Can I see you alone, I don't want to talk on the phone, I need to speak to you urgently," the counsellor said; "I've spoken to his doctor and you are in danger, The Beast has decided a date that he'll be dead. It's going to be messy, he's talking about knives, we are really worried and concerned for all your lives."

'How can he cause harm?'" thought Jane as she drove back to her children, "He's living with his much-beloved mother. Surely the kids and I are safe in our own home." She shook her head and tried to reassure herself that all would be well, that the worse was over, that they were safe.

But as she opened the door, she smelt him, feral, fetid, rabid. Her stomach churned and tightened, her gorge rose, her throat closed. Like a spy in her own home, she silently pushed back the kitchen door and listened. Nothing. Drawers all shut, washing up draining where she had left it. Knives all in the chopping block. Nothing broken. Nothing smashed. Slow steps on cold tiles towards the lounge, past the fridge. Then stop. Stare. For there it was, the sign, the dread. Her calendar reminding her of play dates, of birthdays, invaded by a black noose around the date, arrows leading to the words "Dead. All Dead."

He was here. He was in her house. Her mind closed down, went blank, went into screen saver mode, unmoving until a noise from the adjoining garage woke her from her trance, her hands moving of their own tight-white accord to the handle. As the door crept open she saw his shadow in the gloom and slammed the door against his cackle as he jeered and snarled; "I knew you were too stupid to change the locks. I still have my key, I haven't even broken a window let alone the law and there is nothing you can do to stop me. This is my home bitch and I will come and go as I please. I will haunt you with my terrors until you beg me to take your life, until you know that you are nothing without me, until you are smothered in your own blood, pleading for mercy and knowing there will be none."

"Mummy! Mummy! We're home! Grandma has brought us back. What's for tea?" She heard footsteps behind her, flinched and turned to see Rod swaggering towards the children, smirking. She reached, terrified for the boys only to be pushed hard against the worktop as he crouched down to whisper the kids; "It's alright lads, your mum's gone mad and made a mess of the garage, but I've calmed her down and made her see sense. Sorry to leave you with her but I'll be back to see you soon." Ruffling their bemused, confused curls, leering at the not-fooled-much-alarmed Grandma, he slammed out into the night. Ashen Jane called the locksmith there and then, never thinking to call the police, her mother sensing, but not knowing, what had come to pass, she washed hands, laid the table and made some sandwiches for tea.

LIFE STAGGERED and trembled, but Jane continued to put one foot in front of the other, ears sharp, eyes alert, head turning and scanning at all times, quaking and twitching but continuing with the school run, the dash to work and back.

Until the day she walked in, holding hands with her boys, to hear an old song playing on repeat "Every breath you take, any move you make... I'll be watching you." A cold wind blew through the cracks and the splinters of the unhinged and hanging back door. She went no further but gathered up her boys and fled to her brother's where he settled them to children's TV and dug out some old toys to protect them from the adult alarm.

Days passed, the door replaced and reinforced, the windows were chained and her brother had searched nooks and crannies before confirming it was safe for them to go home.

Returning from a normal day, in a normal town, doing normal things, the three arrived home and did normal things before she put her beloved sleepy heads in bed and started her ordinary routine of packed lunches, washing and sorting her clothes out for the morning. Opening her battered, pine bedroom wardrobe, she stepped back and turned to salt, turned to stone, found herself trapped inside her own musculature, unable to function as she saw the slashed and bloodied remnants of her oft worn clothes and behind them, scrawled in thick black shapes; 'When sorrows come they come not single spies but in battalions'.

When she unfroze, she found that she had once again called her valiant brother, who had carried her little angels to his awaiting car, engine running for a quick getaway if needed. She found that he had taken them home and snuggled the children down. She found that she had a cup of tea in her hand and that there appeared to be tears on her face. "Enough," he said. "Yes," she agreed.

And so it was that she went back to her optimistic and unrealistic solicitor, and told him that mediation and Relate hadn't worked and please could he do something more substantial, more robust, more protective in place. The battle moved from walls and wardrobes to documents and courts. She dreaded every new mailing, every new manoeuvre. The Beast wanted the house, the boys, wanted her money, he wanted the whole lot but most of all, her wanted her pain, he wanted her fear, he wanted her suffering. He was succeeding. Her hair fell out in clumps, her ribs jutted like a deserted hut on a storm ravaged hill, her wrists narrowed to lily stalks, her face drew itself inward, trying to hide the sorrow which escaped from her eyes.

But Life continued on its pilgrimage to a hoped-for promised land. Jane and the boys moved to a little maisonette on a small estate. The courts ruled that Rod had the right to see the kids every Saturday morning, no matter what she or her solicitor said.

And so it was, that on one such suburban Saturday, whilst the neighbours were washing their cars and mowing their lawns, Rod arrived and beeped his car horn which sent the boys scampering towards him. Opening the car doors, he quickly locked them in and menaced his way towards Jane, standing behind the half open, not-quick-enough-to-put-on-the-security-chain door. Slamming it into her and her back to the wall The Beast pulled out a knife and held it up tight against her throat and growled; 'This isn't over, I'll fucking kill you, I'll see you dead yet you bitch."

Life picked up her shaking, quaking, sickened, inert form and stood her back onto her own two feet, breathed itself back into her reluctant lungs, forcing her to inhale, forcing her to fight, forcing her to carry on taking steps.

ANE MET TOM at work. Tom was older. Tom was solid and reliable. Tom was kind. Tom moved to a house near to Jane, not wanting to move too fast for the struggling boys. Jane leaned on Tom. Jane liked Tom. Jane even came, slowly, quietly, to trust Tom.

It was Tom who would stand by Jane's side as she answered the door to The Beast. It was Tom who held her as she sobbed watching the twinned domes of the golden-curled boys disappear in The Beast's black saloon, never completely sure when or if they would return.

The Beast disliked Tom touching his property, his missus, his kids. The Beast threw a cricket ball at Tom's head to teach him to keep away. The Beast scratched his key down Tom's car, scarring it. The Beast swore at Tom, threatened Tom and warned Tom off. But Tom's feet stayed firmly by Jane's side.

So then The Beast played harder ball; writing letters threatening them all with slow, painful dissected deaths. The Beast accused Tom of child abuse, calling him a pervert, a kiddy fiddler, a bastard, a cunt, telling the court his tall tales. The Beast accused Jane of being an unfit mother, a slag, a hooker, a whore. Luckily this court had seen it all before, saw straight through The Beast, putting residential and restraining orders in place, leaving the boys with Jane and Jane with Tom and the boys within the weekend grip of the Beast.

Only Jane and Tom protected the boys. Social services didn't get involved. Schools didn't want to know. The Beast's mother took his side and Jane's mother's courage flourished and flowered. The boys grew to love their mother's mum who, without of the shadow of her long-dead-unmissed husband, was sunny, and kind and fun.

But when the boys went to stay with The Beast they went unprotected and alone. They never spoke of what came to pass, they never showed their wounds until many more winters had passed when one cold and windy night, the now-four-adults sat by a fire and pushed cardboard beer mats around a sticky table as the boys spoke.

The boys told their tales of how when they soiled their pants, their big brave dad, would rub their face in their own shit to teach them not to do it again. Of how when he got a new girlfriend, he ignored them and screamed at them to go away. Of how the eldest son had written his dad a letter, sharing his feelings and his hopes that things could be better, reaching out to mend the rift, but how his dad never replied. The tales which were told were fragments of the truth, the fragments they hoped their mother could bear, with her rock, Tom, still holding her hand, still standing by them all, silent and steady. Even these fragments shattered her heart and sundered her spirit, bowing her head to tears.

Life had carried them forward, to grow up and grow older. Jane had gained recognition and success in her field, Tom and she had created a home and the boys had grown to men.

But still Jane carries a life-long-rock-like burden of guilt, shame and remorse for all the screaming-nights, all the bloody-fights, all the disgusting talk, all the silent knives, all the impossible-to-hide bruises, all the neck scarves to cover the strangle marks, all the blood-stained tissues which didn't flush away, for all the tense tea-times, the ruined Christmas mornings, the anxiety, the flinching, their pain. She couldn't save them though she had tried her best to shield them, her shield had been too frail and fragile to hide the Beast's shadow from her best-beloved-sons.

The Beast lived happily ever after with another woman, one more like his mother the boys say. They think she might hit him, that she might insult and pick on him, they notice how his life has been a circle that way.

Jane's life had gyred and cycled from abusive father to abusive spouse, closing in interminably, sucking her in tight. But Life, her unerring partner, had picked her up when she had fallen, pushed her forward when she stood still, had given her courage where there was dread, given her hope when there was despair.

Turning to Life she asked; "Did I break the cycle? Did I do enough?" Life looked her softly in the eye, pointed at her grown-men-children standing loyally by her side, and smiled.

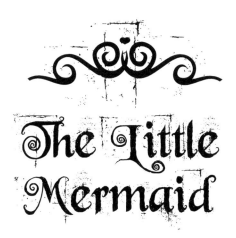

The Little Mermaid

ONCE UPON A TIME there lived a mermaid called Naiad. She lived with her many sisters in the deep blue of the ocean where they would flock and frolic beneath the waves, playing chase with the clown fish who would poke their heads through the rainbow-coloured coral, pulling faces to make the mermaids laugh.

Naiad and her friends loved the days when the pod of dolphins returned from their journeys around the coasts, chasing currents and climates, mackerel and cod. They would peep and pop, calling the teams together before blowing the whistle for the sea-chase of her childhood. Dolphins and mermaids on both teams, dipping and swooping, twisting and twirling, weaving through the sunlit water, whooping and calling to each other as they played.

Playing with the dolphins, it was safe to leap above the waves, towards the sun, into the blue, for the many passing fishermen would look, and rub their eyes, dismissing the girls' turquoise, citrine, coral hair as mere seaweed caught on a dolphin fin, their succulent breasts a trick of the light bouncing on water as the dolphins flew.

Her father Neptune had warned his daughters and his mer-folk many a time about the dangers of tangled nets and hooks, of getting caught in currents that dragged even the strongest tails onto the beach to die. The stories in the mer-school books of her childhood warned of humans and their evil ways; their seduction and temptation, luring young mermaids from their seabeds into beds far rougher and landlocked far away from the oceans. So it was that skyward chase was only allowed under cover

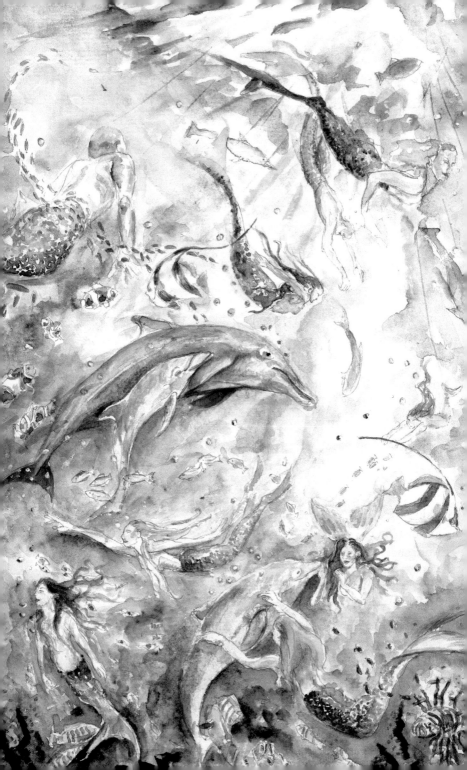

of the dolphin pod or the schools of whales which much more rarely now would return from Arctic and Antarctic seas, so depleted and exhausted from navigating shipping lanes and plastic that they had less energy to play.

Of course the girls had disobeyed their father, as youngsters are wont to do; they had dared each other to hide behind the rocks on bare coves to watch the humans with their awkward legs and silly clothes. Sticking to the shelves of stone with the limpets, draping their tangling, sea-green, purple hair to hide their face, they would watch with amusement at the shoreline squeals of the two-legged, arm waving, wave jumping creatures who seemed so ill-suited for both land and sea.

The adults never glimpsed them, had given up seeing the unseen, had trained themselves to notice only what was expected and to explain away any mystery. But sometimes, one of the younger ones, minds still open to impossibilities, still noticing every grain, every ripple on the sand, would find their eyes and hold their gaze, with curiosity then glee, before running up the beach to tell their disbelieving parents, who would slowly crush their dreams.

Neptune was a kind and distant father, whose mind was on the Seven Seas and so his attention often skimmed like a stone over the surface of the girls' world, rarely sinking in to take a deeper look. Naiad's mother had been a river nymph, not one of the mer-folk at all. There had been much suspicion at her parents' meeting and mating, the other mer-families were wary of her mother's pull towards the rivers and the lakes, not wanting their own merlings to leave the safety of the deep. At mer-school the other merlings soon got used to her two webbed fins, so unlike the singular, powerful tails of her siblings and her peers, not quite as powerful, yet agile and spritely. Her mother honoured her marriage word and never left the deep, although Naiad always sensed a sadness in the way her mother would watch the sun seep into the sea.

Her mother's bedtime stories were tales of distant shores and love, of rivers winding through corn-filled fields and lakes resting in the cradle of soaring peaks and glistening snow. There was magic in the rivers where the beavers built their houses of sticks, where the salmon leaped up stream, and the azure dragonflies wove their spells over brooks on sunny languid evenings whilst the swallows swooped and skimmed to quench their thirst. The humans in these stories were not the hooked and catching ogres of her father's warnings, but barefoot children splashing on sun-gilded pebbles with picnics on the grassy banks, or solitary fishermen, more intent on time alone to mull and lament than on catching anything to eat.

Naiad and her sisters loved their mother, her silken current of rippling mane, her close caresses and listening ear, she was ever present and ever dear. Her daughters had grown into mer-women on the outside, but she still had many years of wisdom to impart when the moon whispered her name and opened up the silvered path, calling their mother home to the sea beyond the sky, out of reach from their pearling eyes and their sundered hearts.

And so it was, on one such full mooned night, that Naiad heard the tides within her stirring and turned to the stars for guidance, following their direction without care for compass or current, through Trafalgar into Fitzroy, ignoring the temperatures falling as she entered Sole, then Fastnet, entering the murk of Lundy , then on, through the mist, into the Irish sea. As if drawn upstream, she glided over the estuarine mudflats, flowed past the rusty chains of anchored crafts, before finding some reeds to curl up in exhausted and lost.

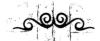

TARTLED, SHE AWOKE to feel her skin tingling and dry where the river had slowly washed her towards an inlet of mud and mossy stones. No mermaid could tolerate this mulched and rotting watercourse, but she, half river nymph, although not at ease, felt not so strange there. Dazed she watched as moorhens busied themselves with their housework and river rats scurried indignantly by, irritated at this confusing fish smell crossing their habitual riverside path.

As she twirled her fingers in the eddies, letting the water boatmen scoot over her submerged stomach, she smiled as she watched the sun rise over fields, not of blue, but green, and watched the pinking of the storybook trees and the gilding of the drops of fairy-tale dew. These were not imaginings after all, what her mother had told her was true. Delighted she watched the swans guide their cygnets from their nests and the heron, iconic in its stilled poise. She felt closer to her mother here, it made her heart hurt less to feel the grass her mother's childish fingers had felt and to breathe the corn-scented air, hearing beasts low and bleat beyond her ken.

She watched with curiosity as a human male wondered down towards the river bank, carrying only a single fishing pole . She saw him sit cross-legged on the grass, before puzzling over hook and line and casting it adrift. She noticed his sun-worn skin and furrowed brow. She had never seen male legs so close before and marvelled at their sinews and their wires.

She watched him in amusement from her hiding place in the rushes as he pulled his line time and time again from the brook, empty. "Be careful," warned the frog, "he'll see you." But Naiad was so entranced she didn't listen. "Be careful," warned the adder as it warmed itself on a nearby stone, "he has hooked others such as you and taken them home." She laughed. He couldn't even catch a minnow let alone one so worldly and well-travelled as she.

She watched as the sun peaked in the sky before turning towards home and bed and continued to peep as she plucked idly at weed, feeding a non-existent appetite that seemed sated just with him in her sight. "Be careful," honked the Canadian Goose, so smart in his evening wear, escorting a swan home, "he's trouble. We've met his type before." She nodded and politely ignored him, she who had swum with the great whales of the oceans and played hide and seek deep in the sea, what had she to fear?

She watched as the man put his head in his hands and sighed at another empty hook and felt her heart ping with pity for the poor man, all alone with nothing to eat. "Be careful," hooted the owl as he swept low, fluttering her hair, "he looks innocent but isn't." What would one so old know of the courage of the young she thought decisively, ducking into the darkening middle of the river and darting her silvered hand out to catch a fish before quietly, and with great care and grace, placing it upon his hook and swimming unseen back to her hiding place.

She watched as the man pulled the silvered shape into the rising moon, happy with his catch. Watched as he pulled a knife from his pocket, and unzipped the fish, letting the guts fall steaming onto the river bank and then pushing them into the stream. She watched as he wrapped her gift with care and tucked it under his arm and set off into the darkening wood.

And so a pattern formed. Each day the man would come to fish. Each time his hook would fail until nightfall when Naiad would reach into the current to provide him with his dinner, unseen, unknown, bursting with desire and curiosity. "Beware," warned the pike, "he'll cause you pain." That's rich coming from a duckling murderer she thought and moved away in disgust.

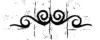

SHE WATCHED for six days, saw how deftly he fitted the hooks, how patiently he waited for his catch, how ruthlessly he would slit the still-pulsing throat of the fish she had guiltily placed there. She had seen the ripple of his muscles beneath his skin, seen him mop the midday sun from his brow, seen him push his ebony hair back with neatly-cut nails and scarred hands. On the seventh day she took her chance. As she hooked the flapping fish onto his lethal barb, she allowed her eyes to break the waterline and find his gazing, without surprise, into hers. "Never," said her father's voice, deep inside her brain, "never let a human male see you alone, for no good has ever come of it." You married mother, she thought in defiance, no one approved of her, she was a different breed and yet what beautiful children you had, I am your child, I will not let love know any bounds.

And so it was that on day eight, she peeped and saw her gaze returned with a smile. On the ninth day, he called to her, called her his water sylph, his diadem, his queen. "Be careful," squeaked the vole, "stay hidden, he's not safe. Go home." Don't tell me what to do you timid, tiny creature you, thought Naiad and plaited her sea-scape hair with poppies and cornflowers humming softly to herself. He no longer arrived so early, and when he did, he would sit and watch, barb and line by his side, resting, waiting, knowing she would come, knowing she was hooked.

On day thirteen she took a breath, and as the sun set its worried head into the cornfields behind, she caught her offering in her silvered shaking hand and swam boldly towards the bank where the brown man sat waiting, assured and poised, still, coiled and ready to receive her willing hand.

They talked long into the night, he sitting on the darkening bank and she in the shallows, hair turning mauve in the setting sun, covering her like a hazy cloak, her finned feet hidden in the moonlit waters. She shared her tales of tickling octopus nannies who could manage any brood, of angel fish and coral, of the pearls and bioluminescence decorating her home.

He told her a tragic tale of childhood hardship, of a fierce and frightening father who would beat before talking, who would shout before asking. She told him about how she and her sisters would taunt and poke the puffer fish just to see it bloat and float and he told her how he and his brothers would run and hide quaking from their father's tread. She told him of her mother's last journey along the moon-road to the sea beyond the sky, of her broken heart, her missing song. He told her about his escape from the childhood battery to faraway lands where he had looked and looked for love finding none, until she.

Her heart twinkled, her lungs sighed, her fins fluttered in excitement. So it was true, all her mother's stories of love at first sight, which also taught how love would conquer all. So as the river passed her by, tugging at her fins to move on, she held on daily to the bank, then his hand until slowly, she moved from the current onto solid land where he curled his nut-brown arm around her silvered skin and held her close, not noticing that her feet still dabbled in the flow. "Escape now, while you can," twitched the rabbit but Naiad ignored its cowardly imploring.

At first he brought her a dress to wear, a startling vermillion-scarlet which hurt her eyes and reminded her of the deadly lion fish before she pushed the thought away. It hurt her tender, undressed skin to have such fabric press so tightly against her hips and breasts and to find her back tied so firmly in. And there was too a tingling, a rising for desire as he stroked the fabric taut against her skin, yet unrecognised for her mother had not grown old enough to name and explain to her the power which lay between her thighs.

Next he brought her tiny transparent triangles of what seemed at first to be the finest black sea-weed that had drifted to the shore. As he explained how to put them on, her heart sunk, now he would see her feet, her fins, her silvered fans, so unlike his solid, fat phalanges, wiggling in the mud.

At first he gasped, and then he laughed and her face flushed with shame as he touched them and stoked them and then smelled them without recoil. "Can you walk?" he asked, and the truth was she didn't know, never having tried. He reached his arms around her and lifted her as she wobbled and wavered and struggled to find her feet. At first she balanced on fin tips, but could find no purchase, no balance, no equilibrium always leaning first this way and then that.

So slowly she pressed down and folded her fins, flattening them onto the solid earth. Thus lily-footed she hobbled her first burning steps, leaning against his sinewed trunk and turning away from the pearls of pain which rolled down her face. His pleasure was her payment, his delight her dowry. She watched as he almost tenderly knelt down to kiss her fins, holding the transparent triangles so she could step in one agonising step at a time. He slowly pulled the un-coverings to the place where her legs met, where the fire changed to lava, and brushed his careless-careful fingers against a place she had never found before.

Tangled with the tendrils of pain and desire, unsure of either, having felt neither before, there on the river bank she succumbed to his tongue across her hips, her thighs as she arched to reach it. His mouth on her neck, biting until it nearly hurt and yet not quite, his fingers grazing her nipples, careless of who could see, hard peaks, sparking waterfalls of wetness in her unexplored cave. Humid, moist, a storm-cloud of desire, predatory, dangerous, unexplored, fascinating. She could not resist the clitoral tingling drawing her to him, his skin, his smell, his eyes, his hair, dissolving will in sucking, gripping, releasing and flowing over and over away from herself as if she were a stream.

It had to be love.

"No, no, no, no!" shrieked the crow, the carrion clarion wise to the forces of life and death, "Leap now, back into the current and re-find your tribe, your pod, your life!" but her mind was too fogged with pain, her ears too clogged with his sweet words of desire to hear. She didn't notice the blood smearing her thighs, matching her harlot garb. Numbed. She could not feel the blistering fins, shedding scales of silver as she struggled to find her feet.

HE HOBBLED her to his tower block home, with his hook firmly packed away until the next time he needed to go fishing. There he dyed her azure-emerald hair, and showed her how to cream her skin to tone away her silver and make her blend in. He bought her jeans which chaffed and rubbed at her tender flesh, tied her fins taut in trainers, binding and encasing them, folding them in on each other, pulling tightly to break the scales and lock her in. He explained to her about food, about fridges, about cooking, about sheets. He explained how to clean the floors, how to iron and scrub. She, an eager student, wanting to please, learned quickly, her heart leaping at his smile, at his approval, at his desire.

Then he went out. She wasn't sure where. He didn't tell her.

So in this hard, concrete casement, high above the grey, grid of her new world, she polished and cleaned, washed and wrung, wiped and chopped all the time ignoring the fire rising from her feet, reminding her how out of her element she was. Ignoring the ache in her heart for how lonely she was. Ignoring the silence in her ears where the sounds of the sea, and the earth and the beasts had been.

Then he would come home and lick her neck, and grip her waist and insinuate himself into her, piercing her ever more deeply.

Slither, writhe. Forget about his temper.

Gasp, grip. Forget that you don't know where he goes.

Suck, lick. Forget that you're all alone.

Shudder, quake. Forget his lies.

Scratch, pull. Ignore that when you go out, he holds onto you so tightly that it hurts.

Groan, sigh. Ignore how he hides from the police, ducks down side roads when their uniforms cross the street.

Poor fisherman, victimised, picked on, a pariah. Only she would understand, only she could make him whole, with her love, only she could heal him from the false accusations with her love, only she could save him.

So she ignored it all and set about saving him as her mother's folk tales had prepared her to do.

UNTIL SOMETHING CHANGED. First, she felt sick, then she felt faint, then her heart burned, then she grew tired, then her breasts swelled, then her skin tensed until finally she wondered, she pondered, she worried, she marvelled that she was carrying a new life in her womb.

So excited she was that she didn't care to look at the kind of father he would be. She dreamed of her childhood birth place, where the merwomen stroked the new mother's skin with unguents and combed her newly lustred hair, singing songs of welcome to the new life inside. She dreamed of the joy and awe the whole reef would feel as the new mer-life joined their tribe, as it was tenderly passed from hand to fin, bestowed with kisses, wishes, and loving-kindness.

She loved how the fisherman would stroke her swelling belly, talking to the life within, and ignored his absences. She loved how he wove promises of the life this new family would live and so didn't notice that it was he who had his feet up whilst she shopped and carried and cooked. She loved how he promised that he would walk through flame and ice to keep his brood safe from harm and so didn't mind, or even notice, that he didn't let her go to the doctor. She ate well for the baby. She got fresh air for the baby but forgot to look after herself. She excused and explained and understood why he slept so late as she heavily staggered from bed to the shops and back. Her baby needed a father and she needed a man, her man to raise this next of kin.

O WHEN THE MEN in blue came to take him away, for reasons to her still unknown, confused by how they searched her rooms and took his hooks, which decorated the wall above their bed, all she knew was that she had to save him, save the father of her child, stand by her man, by her love.

She fought.

She petitioned.

She filled in forms.

She argued.

She travelled this way and that on fins afire with a kicking womb through a land of straight lines, and fast cars and grey faces, all alone.

She spoke to this person and that.

She made this point and that.

'No. No. No'

So, she ordered more papers from here and papers from there, all the time waddling, and leaking, back aching, fins swelling, bump growing, feet pushing, playing tag across the skin between them.

"You should have your feet up"

"Take it easy"

"Focus on the baby"

"Sit down"

"Rest"

Said the official people, said the papermaker-court-keepers, just before they said "No" again.

Like Romeo and Juliet torn asunder, she was Friar and Nurse to their true love's course, galloping after papers here, solicitors there, for she needed her man and her baby needed a father.

When at last the final papers arrived, furled in purple ribbon, sealed in black wax, her heart fluttered; she had worked and won, this would be the document to save her man.

Fingers fluttering, heart trembling, nails inserted under the wax, click-snapping it apart. Unroll the scroll, eyes scanning, pause.

Throat tightening, bile rising, eyes refocusing, heart hammering, mind slowing, hands shaking, teardrops falling, mind closing, paper rolling, paper falling, wax smashing, heart breaking, baby panicking, mother retching.

Women, like she, on hooks.

"It wasn't my fault,'" he would later say. He said they'd lied. The legal teams had lied. The police had lied. It was all a lie. He had suffered, a caged fisherman in his cell, watching the white dove fly free when he was snared in an unfair gaol; misunderstood, suffering in a world that didn't understand him. Always other people lied. Always someone else's fault, always someone telling lies about poor old innocent him.

Prison.

Falling down and down the rabbit hole, spinning, clutching for something to ease her falling, screaming inside so she didn't wake her womb-clothed-babe. Landing with a bump Naiad saw that she had drunk from a potion making her smaller, so tiny she couldn't reach the key to the door to escape.

HEN THE FIRST squeezes came, too early and so were ignored. Sleep, toilet, back to sleep. And then again. And again. 'It can't be' said her head; 'it's too soon. I'm not ready'. But her body was. Her baby was and carried on regardless of her sadness and pain.

Let us stop here and consider the urbane, ubiquitous bravery that birthing is, the 'after' following 'happy ever'. Let's put it in the story now and leave it there. Not the flowers and the cards, not even the pre-morning sickness, the stretching, itching, peeing or the post sagging, scaring, discharging and bleeding. But birth itself. The twisting, squeezing, gripping pain that not only caught her breath but stopped it. No wonder they gave her gas and air – it was to remind her to breathe when stopping would have been the easy option, so tempting.

Let's sing a blood-sister-song to celebrate the women who birth us, birthed you. Stretched, torn, bloodied, drugged. She would have died without the aid of the people in white. Her eyes rolled back, her face turned grey, her lips went blue and frothed. Never tell me that women who birth are not brave, never tell me that, it is not true.

Alone save for the pulsing life within, and then without, she birthed a daughter slimed, bloody, squashed and perfect. Perfectly breathing. Perfectly crying. Perfectly moving. How soon we overlook the miracle that creation is. She would lie in bed and watch her daughter breathe in Hallelujah pose; arms raised in celebration, fists curled, legs bandied, oblivious and milky. She would marvel at her pouty lips, her bluish eyelids, her downy hair and she would forget that she too was born perfect. Not perfectly beautiful or perfectly gifted or perfectly graceful, just perfectly herself.

And so gazing at the baby, her baby, she did not see mirrored in her child her own perfection; she saw only her inadequacies; never feeling good enough, not up to the job. And we never are perfect parents, just good enough, if we are lucky. She gave birth to her new self; a mother and a father to this fingerling, she would build a new life for the fisherman to join them in.

She loved this child, she loved her curly hair, her cheeky smile, her smell. To feel her breathing, to reach out and feel her, warm and sleeping.

Did her daughter need skin to skin or did she? She would look back at this time as Eden, as golden, as paradise lost. The two of them, happy, playing, laughing.

She left the bricks and blocks, the stairs and stones and moved to a sturdy hut, by a stream, strewn with the detritus of uncaring hands, behind the waterworks, where at least she could see the setting sun across the disused scrub of wasteland. She released her fins from their bindings and allowed them to feel once more the damp joy of oozing mud. She let the dye fade from her cornflower hair and her skin once more shone like silver stars.

These were happy times. The day-to-day miracles of smiling, crawling, walking, talking, singing, playing, hiding, seeking, tickling, reading, imagining. The sun was out and the ground was warm and steady as they baked the fish she caught and made bubbles and played tag with the dragonflies who always won. They snuggled and snoozed and wandered the welcoming banks, slowly cleaning away the waste they found, making friends with their froggy neighbours, the cautious voles and the ducks.

Her daughter took naturally to water, she would splash and paddle, throw rainbows of jewelled drops from her small hand to Naiad's and loved to bob in her warm arms, held in the shallows, watching their reflections, happily connected and reflected in the water and the sky. She was not, she noticed sadly, of mer or Naiad blood fully filled, for although she loved to kick and float, she had not her mother's lungs of water and of air, had not her fins, had not her silvered skin, would never see the prisms of light illuminated plankton, the coral-floral crannies, the waves of nickel coated tuna, nor play catch with the porpoises in Cape Cod.

SHE CLEARED and mothered, and fished and mothered, and played and mothered and papered and petitioned and lawed and fought for the fisherman and then fished and cleared and mothered some more.

All this she did because she knew a baby needs a dad and a woman needs a man and that woman stands by her man no matter about the hooks.

She sent him the pennies scrabbled from her riverbank recycling.

She painted pictures for him of their daughter.

She saved her coins to make brief calls, only allowed at certain times, always listened to by the guards.

His cell was too far away for her to visit, she didn't have the means or wealth so instead she contacted charities, advisories, anyone who might help.

Meanwhile he fought in a different way,

Hurt someone else.

Only once he would later say,

But she never believed him again.

What was he to do, poor man, he was being picked on, the other man deserved it.

Now he had an extended stay.

And when she couldn't forgive and forget, it was all her fault.

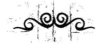

AT LAST HE DID return to meet her nearly-school-age talking-toddler in her little cabin on the edge where the river met the land.

Now they could live happily ever after.

Phew.

She bound her fins again.

Dyed her hair again.

Covered her silver again.

Found work for him.

Did his washing for him.

Shared her pennies with him.

Shared her home with him.

Her bed with him.

She tried to share her body with him but her body said 'no', even when her mind said 'I should'. There is nothing like giving birth to give a body a voice, but loud though hers was shouting about disgust and revulsion, her head still spoke louder with vows and duties and shoulds.

And all the while she forgot to take care of herself and he certainly wasn't.

First the shouting started.

Then the slammed doors.

Then the disappearances.

Then the blaming.

Then the lying.

Then the denials.

Of course it wasn't him who nearly burned the house down by leaving the fire unattended; it must have been her fault.

It was her fault that he put his hand through the window, how dare she ask where he was going?

It was her fault that the chair got thrown across the room breaking the light, telling him what to do!

It was the daughter's fault for not doing what she was told, that's why she got screamed at.

It was the bank's fault that they closed his account.

It wasn't his fault that her furry and reptilian friends stopped coming around, it was his hut now and he didn't have to talk to them.

It wasn't his fault that he lost his jobs, they were ripping him off, treating him unfair.

It wasn't his fault that she never went out just because he'd told her she looked fat or stupid in whatever she was wearing.

It wasn't his fault he didn't take care of their daughter whilst she was out clearing the river flotsam. So what if he'd agreed? He'd forgotten.

It was her fault that she couldn't get over his hooks and his fighting.

It was her fault that their daughter hid from him.

It was her fault they were poor, she should be earning more.

Her once ruddy, smiling, chubby, curling happy girl, started to awake screaming from bad dreams and was scared to be alone. Naiad preferred to leave her with the mother duck while she combed and cleaned the river's course, even though the father was at home, feet up, unemployed, her daughter was safer with the she-duck and her brace.

Her daughter started to cough and choke, struggling to breathe in the eggshell atmosphere, strangled by her father's glares and scowls, fearful as she cowered behind his shielding mother, holding her hem like a talisman to ward off evil spirits.

The best of times were when Naiad and her daughter were alone or playing with the river folk, making friends, with rat and mole. She overcame the daily betrayals, the unexplained absences, the moods, the nights she went to bed wondering if she would wake up.

TILL SHE CARRIED ON. Until one morning, her flippered feet, yet to be bound, her sliver skin, glowing between the made-up smudges, she stepped into where her daughter was playing with the acorns and pine cones the squirrels had gifted her, to see the fisherman's fist raised high, bearing down on her beloved, so small and young. Frozen in time, burned into her still, fist raised, face of thunder, closing in. To see such a threat; tigress reactions, she stood between then gathering her girl fled to the swans across the river who, when the fisherman came demanding his daughter, reared up with outstretched wings and sent him scuttling away.

Naiad didn't know she should call the police, didn't know it would have protected them to have at least a note on file. Instead she took her daughter to school and went to her river-work. She told them all about the furious raised fist and the cowering small child but no one, not one soul, said; "Phone the police." Not one of them said; "Your child is at risk." Not one of them said; "Are you scared? Does he do this a lot?" Yes and Yes.

Standing alone to protect her child she told him not to come home, not after what he had tried to do.

But when, that night, her daughter asked where daddy was, her torn heart and confused head let him back in, on the condition of three tasks; that he go to parenting classes to learn some different ways than thumping, that he go the doctor to get help for his anger, that he talk to three Riverside men about what he'd done, so they could tell him how to behave.

So he charmed his way through parenting classes, the perfect dad, charming the other mothers with his tales of playing and helping whilst ignoring the worn-out and trembling Naiad.

He charmed the doctor who proclaimed he didn't have an anger issue, he was just really stressed.

He charmed three Riverside men, who said that trying to thump your kid wasn't really how we water-way men do things old chap.

No one said; "Trying to thump you kid is child abuse."

So home he came.

Only one Grandmother from the parenting course had the courage to see what was in front of her and speak her truth, sending Naiad a message in the blackbird's beak; 'There is nothing wrong with your parenting, it's your marriage that is the problem'.

At which point Naiad's head went pop; a ball of white light exploded from within, scattering shards of sun-spark all over the kitchen floor, where she scrabbled and grabbed for them, wailing and muttering like a lunatic.

Blank.

Blank.

No thoughts.

Nothing.

No work.

No river.

No house-holding.

No mothering.

Nothing but flesh flailing against wall and floor.

He drove her sobbing and shaking to the doctor who knew about the intended punch but said nothing. Who proclaimed her stressed and signed her off work and told her to rest.

Home she went and screamed, sobbed, rocked, banged her head, pulled her hair, thumped the wall, unbound her feet and scratched the makeup from her silver until the blood showed through the pewter of her tarnished skin. Locking herself in the toilet so no one would hear and take her away, or worse, take her daughter away from her.

If the madness leaked out when her girl was near, she fought against it and sometimes lost. The girl brought her mother her teddy and gave her hugs. The shame of how she must have terrified her small daughter was greater than the pain as she pulled out her dyed hair, thumped the walls and smashed her head over and over on anything that was hard, any pain welcome.

Screaming at the fisherman she wailed; "Why don't you just hit me and get it over with?" The torment of the lies and the leaving and the impending threat was suffocating and she knew that if he hit her then she could leave. But of course he didn't hit, that was too easy, too obvious, he had learned the hard way that crime doesn't pay but oh manipulation, fabrication, confabulation were skills and magic which could slowly, slowly eat away at the mind, leaving only the body as a screaming shell.

She repainted the hut sunset orange. She had needed to see change. There needed to be change. But before such thoughts could form there was blanking, sobbing, hurting, bashing, lying alone on the scrubbed wooden floor, sprawled, tearing pages, scribbling in crayon, black, red, orange, pushing so hard the pages tore.

AND YET, through it all, another part of her, quiet and small, watched and knew it would all be OK. Knowing that it was a necessary breaking apart, breaking away, breaking down of all that she had held on to, all the dreams and fairy stories needed to come tumbling down. There was some relief in her stilled mind. Only in breaking, shattering, fragmenting could she find the quiet, whole peaceful place inside her. As she slowly, slowly got up off the floor and jigsawed herself back together, she put herself back in the picture. Made herself part of the equation.

She unbound her feet and threw away the dulling cream that crusted her skin. She allowed her blue roots to peep through the dead, dark dye that had held its radiance at bay for too long. She started to swim again, to join the swans and moorhens in the river's flow, floating more. The water of the river suspending her, holding her even as she cried. She thanked the waters as she fell in, thanked them for always being there, silently accepting, allowing her to be exactly as she was no matter how up or down she felt. Rebirthing her every time. Introducing her to her body cold cell by cell. Allowing the cracks in her soul to heal and encouraging the ball of white light to roll down her spine, through her flesh and bones, diffusing every neuron, every sinew, every lash and hair. For only when we are truly broken can the light flood in.

And the lightholders came with their gifts, the gruff old badgers with their immaculate morning coats, the river rats, quick and smart, survival their art, the heron with her poise and grace, the trout that tickled her unfurled fins as she and her daughter paddled in the shallows. They gifted her with reminders of their love, helped her see her reflection clearly in the brook, see her worth and her courage. They tangled feathers in her hair to remind her she was free to fly. They cloaked her in meadow flowers to remind her that there was always growth, always blossoming, even in the harshest soil. They soothed and spread out her folded fins, massaging them with oils and perfumes, easing the contraction of being folded in. They polished her silvered skin with the thistledown and cast-off wool of spring-born lambs, wiping away the years of pretending to be someone else, someone he had wanted her to be. Their circle of light lifted her from the scribbles on the floor until she had the strength to know she didn't need to live in darkness any more.

"It is done," she said simply, with a certainty and finality that he heard and the river creatures stood in still observance as he packed his hooks and left the little wooden cabin on the river banks for good.

Happy ever after.

O R MAYBE NOT. Because the fisherman's greedy half-brother came slouching by, uninvited, unwelcome, trailing smoky resentment in plumes in his wake. He eyed this, priced that, scowled around this corner and muttered into that and span the wheel of fortune upside down and inside out.

At first the fisherman wanted a bite, then the apple, then the apple tree, then the land, the house and all that he could see. He went for the lot, and maintenance, for, she gasped, because she had collected river junk and worked when he had not, she could be called on to support her dependent, who had been too busy hooking other women to find himself a job. The panic washed over her from newly-relaxed fins, past her flailing heart, spinning her head as it coursed through; he would take her home; the log cabin on sturdy legs. He could make them homeless. He would do that to his daughter. He was allowed to do that. Incredulous.

Pennies went missing from her daughter's money box, doors opened without permission, her nightgowned girl dragged into cold nights and all the while she worked and mothered, doing neither as well as she would have liked.

The eggshells were cracked but not yet broken, until one day, collecting her daughter from school he turned – screaming, shouting, following her home, trying to drive off with the girl, doors open, toddler toppling. The mighty river-folk circled to protect the child and keep them safe. Police were called, locks being changed when he forced his way across her threshold, fearful for her life "You need to go... You need to go..." Broken record... "You need to go."

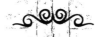

SLOWLY LIFE THAWED. They awoke from their sleep and started to stretch. Her shoulders dropped, the tension melted from the house. She breathed fully once more. Her jaw unclenched. The guilt, oh the guilt of being mother and father too, of missing Harvest Festival and the time off work when her girl was ill. Guilt: mother's little torturer, never far away; the shadow-like stalking of the impossible story of having it all, being it all, without it all falling apart because the centre cannot hold.

And yet, juggling and working was worth it, because when it had been time to start her life anew without him in tow, she could feed her daughter, pay the bills, put a roof over their heads; and when, for the months she feared he would take it away, she resigned herself to living in a tent, her tent, with her freedom and her friends; so much better than living with him. Safe. No hooks.

It was only after the papers were signed and their home was truly safe, many moons later, that they were released from the dark of the dread. And in the dusty, grubby, children's-pictures-peeling-from-from-the-walls kitchen, sipping water and talking in a circle of women, hens, does and pens, Naiad tried to explain to their confused faces why she wasn't happy to let her getting-bigger-yet-still-too-small girl stay overnight with her father.

It was only as she explained how scared she was, how her daughter was frightened by his abrasive, sulky, foreboding ways, that a world-wisened woman said "Domestic violence." Blinkered, startled, she bucked and shied away.

"Oh no!" she said, "But he never hit me or my girl," (because, she thought, I always stood in the way). The words circled her head like crows before taking roost: domestic violence, verbal, emotional, psychological, threat, and control, lying, and more. As the dark shapes settled into their nest; clarity hatched:

The waking up nightly and wondering if she would still be alive to see dawn.

The isolation, the way friends were forced out by his sulking and his tempers; scared away.

The days when he promised to catch her but let her fall backwards, nowhere to be seen.

Calling her mad and hysterical and an unfit mother.

Calling her frigid or a slag or saggy and old.

Hiding money.

Telling stories.

Denying the obvious.

Taking away her solid ground.

Chip. Chip. Chip.

T'is common, she would later find, sitting in another ring of women, doing the therapy, reading books.

The naming of it was powerful, the label contained and shaped it, made sense of the crying kitchen floor. How far out of her element she had been, how high and dry hooked into his land, the spiralling, maze-like conversations that always ended up back at her fault.

And then started the grief and recrimination, the self-blame, the judging, the shame and the pain. 'How can I have been so stupid, so gullible, so blinded. How did I get into this mess? How was I so powerfully entranced?'.

ONE MORNING as the sun twinkled the dew over breakfast she saw a small dark jot fall from the elder bough. Leaving her girl playing she went to watch and watch and watch the dark dot of a moth wiggle and squirm and throb and rest its way from its cocoon. She wanted to rescue it, help it, hurry it, protect it... and yet she could do, would do, nothing but witness its struggle to change and grow to free itself from the self-made constraints of the cocoon. Comfortable and protective yet constricting and suffocating. For at last she understood that the webs that bound her were her own making, her own spells woven of old. She, moth-like, would wiggle and struggle season by season to ease herself free, bit by bit to join the blue vastness and for the first time fly free.

Slowly she began to unravel the stories of good girls, good mothers and good wives, and being nice and keeping quiet and keeping everyone else happy before herself. As she sat on her wobbly wooden step one bright day, she saw a red kite circle overhead, playing with the thermals, arrowed tail direct and clear against the white scuds of cloud. "Sister," it called, "you have given your daughter roots, now let her see your wings, your fins. Let her see you float high and free. Let her see how you both can soar and swoop and play."

So she taught her daughter to swim further out, further downstream each day until they reached the mouth where the river met the sea and where the land fell away into the vast expanse of sky. There she taught her girl to find her strength and stroke, to navigate the currents, the tides, the waves. She learned to read the faces of the moon, to steer by the stars, to find the thermohaline circulation, to read the Coriolis effect.

When the girl grew tired she would rest her head upon her mother's breast and sleep, her green hair swirling round them in the brine. Sometimes she would whistle to the whales who would bear her daughter aloft for a while, to draw her breath whilst she flicked her fins and joined them in their undulations across the sea-scape. The girl joined with the pods of dolphins in the setting sun, keeping goal, unable to follow them into the depths, but enough of a water child to play. Her mer-sisters loved their niece and Neptune welcomed her as one of their tribe, even though her roots were more earthy than their own.

And so it was that Naiad and her daughter lived between the worlds of the land and the sea, of the river and the meadow, of the seen and the unseen, returning to their beloved hut with their river folk after exploring the unfathomable sea.

And on a full moon, with her daughter tucked safely in her walnut bed, watched over by the owls and vixen, you might see Naiad flip from the shallows into the deep, downstream to the wide open arms of the sea, where she joins her sisters somersaulting in the moon path, singing moon songs to their mother, to the mothers of the world, whether land, sky or sea, that wherever, whoever they are, they may all be loved, safe and free.

Jack and the Beanstalk

JACK AND JILL WENT up a hill, to fetch a pail of water,
Jack fell down,
And broke his crown,
And Jill came tumbling after.

Jill lived with her mother and father at the foot of the hill, in the wide spaces of the meadows, where the skies were often blue and the skylark's song accompanied Jill's childhood. She muddied her knees in puddles, collected rose petals for jars of perfume and knew her bluebells from her primroses, her blackberries from her sloes. She had much time to stand and stare. Jill was free to go and play with lambs in spring, collect acorns in autumn, watch as the squirrels hid their nuts in grass, and form snowmen in the winter. She biked the back lanes, the gentle wind tugging at her kinky hair, tickling it into her eyes. She saw daylight streams full of stars, she hid and sought her friends, she was fast to tag and slow to quit, her laugh came easily.

Beyond the meadow was a sombre, dark and creaking wood, of tripping ivy and snagging brambles, where she imagined bears making dens. Her friends and family never went in there, and although no one ever told her not to, why would she ever venture forth when the meadow was so light, bright and free?

Her mum loved her dad and her dad loved her mum and she grew up in a happy home. Her father searching and seeking, moved from a fire-and-brimstone, halleluiah church, of sinners-and-saints, to a quietly spoken Quaker meeting house where Jill's teenage years were filled with friends and sharing: sharing time, sharing food, sharing fun and thoughts; acceptance was the password and tolerance was the key. There was good and God in everyone and forgiveness was the liturgy;

Forgive us our trespasses as we forgive those who trespass against us.

Jill was a feisty lass who fought for the underdog; collecting social issues to champion; marching for CND; fighting for equality – safe and secure in her loving home. Her parents were proud of her cloak of courage and encouraged her to be a force for good in the world, and she was.

As puberty passed and teenage spots settled into a blooming glow, Jill began to stretch her legs and lengthen her view. She wanted adventures, she wanted to fight dragons, to rescue the oppressed and to heal the sick. But the meadow was too flat and tame. It was always the same. The seasons would come and go, and although the meadow was beautiful it was boring, nothing exciting ever happened there.

One golden day when Jill was overheating in the sun, a small breeze ran up her reclining spine, and whispered into her ear, 'The wood, the wood, we should explore the wood'. Jill took a breath, shook the flurry out of her ears and considered for a moment, unsure. None of her tribe had ever ventured beyond the cornflowered and poppied pleasantries of the grasslands, she had no compass or map and was unsure of how or if to sally forth.

IT WAS A RUBIED butterfly that drew her forward, flittering her attention across the corn-tops and the stiles and leading her towards the twisted woodland paths. Stepping out of the sun's glare, into the greenwood shadow was a welcoming caress of cool. She didn't notice the butterfly turn once more towards the sun, nor did she hear the harsh cawing of the nesting crows; she was seduced by the succulent sod, its dewy moisture bathing her parched feet.

She stood a while in thought, looking down the two paths she saw ahead through the wood. One was hardened mud, cracked into earthy paving slabs, wide enough to proceed without being scratched or scraped; straight and clear. The other, more undulating and confused called her with a riot of ramsons, jumbles of foxgloves, delicate celandine and fearsome belladonna; they tempted her with their perfumed promises and she took them at their word.

The half-hidden track led her into the wood. Sometimes her path crossed the well-worn bridleways of pub beer gardens where she would stop for a while, quaffing honeyed mead and oaty ale. Once or twice she found herself alongside highways where people gyrated and span in clubs or gigs where the notes tingled her spine and moved her limbs in most delightful ways. What an exploit! What an escapade! Now she was really living, following her own track and crossing the trails of others, sharing words, episodes, incidents and affairs, living life like the skylark, high and harebell-cobalt-free.

She was no stranger to solitude and welcomed its spacious presence after the jangling of the partied crowds, she had found her feet amongst the sward and was happy to take each step on her own terms, in her own time. It was very rare that anything save rabbits, squirrels or the ebony blackbird joined her on her trail and when the occasional pair of uninvited, alien, sandaled-feet did approach from ahead or behind, she would lower her gaze, sink earthward and simply sit and wait for them to pass, preferring to be alone.

NTIL ONE DAY when some feet stopped in front of her, trainer-toe-tips pointing towards her too-close-now knees. She waited. The feet did too. Her heart began to race, for these feet were in her space; she would have to move. Palms pushing into the soft, mossy, cushion, she leaned forward, elevating herself. She raised her eyes to see bracken brown calves, gnarled knees, a solid trunk, wide oaken shoulders from which fell the boughs of strong arms. Following her eyes to his face, she found there a handsomely soft smile, waiting patiently for her to enter its golden charm. He was gorgeous: translucent, faintly scarred skin, his masculine chiselled jaw, his pools-of-dark-sorrowful eyes, his brow heavy with tragedy; she was intrigued and so let her steps fall in with his; a potential project; someone to rescue.

His name was Jack.

He weaved his tale of wail and woe. His father, previously wed, having produced five bairns, then up and eloped with Jack's mother, bringing her five mouths to feed before having five more of their own. She did the best she could, given that her own mother, Jack's grandmother, had been as mad as a box of frogs. With tragi-comic inevitability, Jack's parents parted ways and he took the road his father trod but was only a tender seventeen when his father dropped his head, dead, on the bed.

Jack blamed himself; he had known his father's heart was weak, he should have carried the loads, driven the car, tidied the house, earned the money and then his father would still be alive. His fault. All his fault and so he had spiralled down, deeper on down into the well of depression, deprivation and drugs.

He had slowly clambered up the wheel of life to find his greatest-love-for-all-time. They soon became betrothed and wedding bells were booked. Until days before the church would open its doors to them, she and her car were shattered and compressed beneath a hurtling lorry. Her beloved heart, bestilled.

Jill's eyes pooled and her arms unfurled to slowly welcome him into her heart-space. She knew that she could save his wounded soul for there was God and good in everyone. She sent the robin with an excited announcement of her new love for her mother; "I have found the man I want to marry." "Stop! Don't!", came the flustered-epistle, via the jackdaw's sharpened claws; "We've asked around, he's not nice, come home at once." "They can't tell me what to do," thought the adventuress, and she stubbornly dug her heels into the grubby, leaf-moulded floor.

"Come with me, to where I live" crooned her sweet man's song; "We can live alone in peace, no one will bother us, I'll share my world with you."

With that, Jack pointed up through the canopy of ochred-terracotta foliage to the stormy, slate-grey, sky. "My castle is in the sky." He simply said, "and you will need these five magical beans to follow me there."

He held out his rugged, bear-like palm where she saw five oxblood, cordovan, curved beans waiting patiently for her.

She picked up one.

Amazed she heard it whisper; "I am the love bean – plant me beneath your feet and feel my love for you grow."

Then she chose a second bean and wondered as it promised; "Plant me and our trust will grow; you will trust me with your life, I will belong to you and stay faithful to you amongst all others."

The third bean made her smile with joy as it assured her; "Plant me and I will protect you from all harm."

The fourth bean reassured her in its resonant timbre; "Plant me and I will take care of you, pay for you, provide a house for you; you will never want for anything."

The final bean sonorously proclaimed; "Plant me and I will give you children, we will share the fruit of our loins and raise them in a loving home."

Taking each small, vibrating bean she knelt down and sunk her fingers into the yielding loam, making a womb for every one, before tucking them in tightly and willing them to grow. She fell asleep in Jack's warm arms, watched only by the anxious, peeking, waning moon, and dreamed of hearts and rainbows and kittens.

It was dark when she woke, and cold, and she was scared to find herself alone. Having joined hands with this strong man, solitude was no longer enticing. At first, she couldn't understand why she was so overshadowed at this late-wood-pigeon-call time of morning. She looked around, but the solid oaks crossed their arms, the resplendent chestnuts shook their reddish heads and the wind-milling-sycamore-scythes cut their way through the air and flew. Then she cast her glance towards the floor and saw the dappled light of late autumn sun was usurped by twilight, nightshade; deadly.

FINALLY, SHE FURROWED her brow and raised her eyes and to her amazement saw, rising high and haughty, a beanstalk. It twisted, serpentine, skyward, pushing and shoving its head through the starlinged horizon. In excited expectation she left her path and fought her way through the wood towards the giant stalk. The elms whipped her arms to hold her back, the brambles snagged her shins to stop her, the mud sucked down her shoes to slow her down and the beech and hazels ganged together forming coppices to stand in her way; but nothing could stop her.

Jack built Jill a stalk by his will
And invited her up to share it

She didn't know
For his evil didn't show
That eventually she would despair it

Her small hands curved around it's silken, slimy, circular stem and she struggled to find a grip. She could see no way to scale its monstrous proportions but knew that she must try. She started to perambulate its rooted girth, scratching and scrabbling, grappling and slipping, cursing and frustrated. Where was Jack and why wasn't he here to help?

"Sorry love," she heard him, slightly slurred, "just had to pop into the Royal Oak to do a bit of business. Jeez you're looking hot today, let's get you up those stairs to bed." Without further ado, he clapped three times and knocked twice on a canker-mark on the mulch-green stalk-trunk. A door sprung open before Jill's eyes and Jack beckoned that she follow.

She stepped inside, without noticing the wailing of the wind in the leaves or the shudder of fear in the earth; only feeling Jack's mouth against her neck calling forth the sap of her desire. "All those stairs," she gasped, surveying the steps spiralling into the baize yonder, "it will take us years to climb them." "Yeah", he agreed, "It would. That's why I've got a lift."

Jack and Jill went up the hill.

Jack tugged at a fleshy tendril and two octopusine, boa-esque tentacles, one for Jack, one for Jill, snaked their way around their flesh and pulled them up and up, through the guts of the stalk before finally depositing them in a uterine, musty, mildewy cavern which seemed bejewelled and bejazzled to Jill.

"WELCOME TO MY HOME" he said. Before devouring her with his swollen lips, stroking her with his burning fingertips, and parting her ways with his tongue. It was later that evening that having supped and satisfied his carnal needs, Jack fetched an old guitar and a brown sack, tied with rough, fraying string. He opened the sack and emptied it onto the scrubbed, wooden table. Jill gasped. She had never seen so many shining golden coins before and reached to stroke and trickle them through her fingers. "Not so soon my dear,"

purred Jack, "First listen to my guitar." As he plucked and picked and strummed, Jill felt woozy, felt foggy, felt far away. Enchanted, she fell asleep, blissfully unaware.

Isolated now, in her castle in the sky, Jill had made her bed and so lay in it, and soon found herself pregnant. Jack would often disappear at moonrise, appearing only at dew-dry, sluggish and intoxicated and stoned. He would thump the hardening arterial walls of his stalk, and patrol the perimeters moodily, keeping Jill safely under his control. The names he called her made her stomach churn, she would clamp her sweating palms to her ears to block out the arrows of disdain and pain, but he would simply twist her wrists away and hurl abuse some more. Whenever she tried to protest or resist he would simply play his guitar and Jill would slump as if drunk, in distant reverie and succumb to his dream.

Alone, Jill would stand on her tippy toes to peek out over the woods to the meadow and her heart shrunk when she thought of all she had left and lost there. She wished she could reach out to her parents, did they even know where she was?

The stalk was too high for the squirrels to climb, too slimy for the beetles to burrow in, too bare for the doves to nest in and too tall for the thrushes to swoop by. Jill was too frightened of the serpentine-tendril lift, and whenever she opened the door to the dizzying stairwell, she would sway with vertiginous fatigue just at the thought of descending step by step. Jill really was stuck and all alone.

As her stomach grew and the baby wiggled and kicked she knew she needed to reach out for help. She realised that the guitar held a magic in its chords which captured her thinking and threw it to the west wind; she was unable to resist it. When Jack played, she was bewitched, entranced and mesmerised. He would shout and storm and humiliate her and then when she crumbled into rivulets of tears, he would play the guitar and seduce her until she fell asleep, and then do it all again.

It was only when Jack was gone that the spell lost its power and she knew what she must do. With secret, underarm cuts, she removed small balls of fleece from her coat's filling and stuffed them into her ears; yes, these would muffle the sound. So that night, after another battering, this time for not having his washing dry on time, as she crunched, sobbing into the corner, Jack brought out his guitar to soothe her to get his wicked, loined way. She heard the melody, but the notes could do no more than waft around her ears, unable to enter, and so soon flew away. She, of course, pretended to be beguiled, and feigned sleep and compliance, but all the time, she was thinking for herself. She knew things had to change.

One day, as she was craning to look out from her high, narrow-arrow-slit windows, she saw a lone bird, much higher than the rest, a buzzard spiralling heaven-ward on the thermals. She watched as tears of freedom-lost traced her bruised cheekbone and her bloodied nose before tripping over her own chin, silly girl. "Buzzard! Mr Buzzard!" She called, "Please fly over here! I need help!" But instead the golden bird drifted away, following unseen currents in his search for prey.

Later that night at supper, which once again hadn't been just to his liking, so he'd rubbed her nose in it before smashing the door on his way out, she salvaged a morsel of meat, which only he was allowed to eat, as money was tight, didn't she know. Returning to the corner of the room where her pallet bed lay, she started to unravel the stitches at the hem of her dress, drawing out a length of thread. Tying the meat to the thread with fumbling fingers, she headed eagerly towards the slithered-slots of the windows straining to spot the buzzard. But he didn't show and she awoke stiff and tired, leaning against the sill, to the sound of the serpent lift returning the father of her child, to his kingdom and wench.

The next day and the next, she leaned and pined out of the sharp-cut-windows, each night, replacing the mouldering meat with some new, until at dusk on the third day she spied the buzzard circling high. "Mr Buzzard! Mr Buzzard! Please fly over here, I need your help!" and she twirled the flesh-fastened thread to draw him to her. Wily and aware, the buzzard caught the meat but hovered still and curious at this creature with the red-rimmed eyes, ringed yellow and green.

"Who are you and what do you want?"

So Jill told him her story and asked; "Please, will you send my word to my mother that my child is due and I need help, let her know where I am and tell her to come quick." The Buzzard felt a curious sensation rising through its gut, tugging on its ribcage and squeezing on its heart. Pity. Was this pity? A sensation new to him; he agreed and she watched him grow smaller and smaller against the fading horizon.

The next morning, whilst Jack was still snoring on his sumptuous-feather-plumbed bed, and Jill was sweeping the cobwebs from his clothes and floor, a siren shouted out; "Intruders! Intruders! Intruders at the house!" Jack leapt from his slumbers with a start and headed to the lift door. She had never noticed the intercom before; the perforations in the stem. "What? What do you want? Who is it? Go away!" Jack screamed.

But Jill's mother, father and the health visitor would not go away, and, wanting to avoid trouble, Jack put on his charming face and welcomed them in, full of apologies for not having known who they were. Jill, too, made excuses for him; "He's not usually like that," she swore, without conviction, her mother saw. And so, it was agreed that Jill would leave the stalk for hospital and baby care and later for work, but only on his terms.

THE GOLDEN-EGG-BABY was born and Jack and Jill wed, because that's what children need; two parents who are married. Jill's grandmother was so pleased, her parents looked wary and drawn at the very small ceremony in a deserted town hall. The groom arrived, staggering, smelling of hops and tar, with a black eye from some bloke who deserved everything he got.

Jack and Jill went up the hill
Jack had wanted a daughter
When he got a lad
He went mad
And beat Jill till she was vomiting after

Golden-egg-baby-boy was only three months old when Jack snatched the suckling babe from its mother's breast, wrapped it in his coarse, horsehair coat and descended the stalk shouting "You have no rights! He's my son!" Frantic, Jill made for the lift to follow but found it locked. She called to her buzzard who was roosting for the night and could not hear. She called to the owls who were too busy honing their stealth to answer her call. She was stuck, high above her path, high out of sight, out of sound; there was nothing she could do but rock and weep and wait.

When Golden-egg-baby-boy started to wail, Jack plonked his son on his own mother's doorstep; "You deal with the squalling brat," he commanded. But sensibly, she persuaded him to return the baby to its mother's arms. Jack fairly flung Golden-egg-baby-boy at Jill before descending to the bars and bras which kept him so amused.

As Golden-egg-baby-boy grew, Jill was allowed out to toddler groups, she even made some friends. Jack got a job and life seemed steady enough. She got used to the timer on the lift, allowing her just enough time to get to work and back before it locked her out. She dare not stay to chat or even return a friendly wave as she knew she wouldn't survive a night out in the forest all alone, unsure if Jack would relent and let her in.

Time passed and Golden-egg-baby-boy-two was born. Jill felt poor, she never again saw the sack of gold coins and made ends barely meet from the family allowance that the postman pushed nervously through the door. Jack started to drink again and Jill got used to hiding the kitchen knives when he was out, so they were not to hand on his staggering return.

Jack and Jill continued still
Jill looked after the babies
Jack liked to beat
And tip Jill out of her seat
Cracking her chin on the table

Once upon a time Golden-egg-baby-boy-two was pulling himself up on his cot-prison-bars. Jack, having just returned from his drinking, grabbed a knife and held it over the baby screaming; "I want you to go! I'm going to have the children! I'm going to tell everyone you're an unfit mother! You need to get out now!" Like a cornered tigress Jill replied; "I'll go, but I'll go in the morning," and in so doing saved her babes from who-knows-what fate, for in the morning Jack could remember nothing and Jill was too scared and relieved to mention it.

Jack was mean and cruel to Jill
He sometimes locked her in the bedroom
He'd hide the key
So she couldn't get free
Or even get out to the bathroom

Once upon another time, when the children were only one and two, Jack strangled Jill so hard that he left red marks around her neck. He threw her out into the iced-January forest on a new moon wearing only her nightie and told her not to bother coming home. Desperate for her children still locked in the stalk, Jill blindly scrambled her way to a woodland wire and made a reverse charge call home to her mum who woke her dad and drove their best-beloved daughter shaking and quaking and bruised to the police station, to find that they were simply not interested. Not one bit. Not at all.

Jill spent that night in a Wood-Travel-Inn and then went home to her Golden-egg-boys.

The Golden-egg-boys grew and grew and Jill thought about home schooling. "Please don't" pleaded her concerned and powerless father. He knew that Jill and the children needed to be out in the woods or the meadows where they would not be so alone. A wise man. Jill listened. But she wouldn't leave her husband. It's not what boys need she thought; they need two parents at home. Everyone knows that.

Jack wanted a third child, but Jill had managed to sneak to the doctors on one of her stalk-prison breaks and begged for the pill. One day Jack found the little white saviours hidden in Jill's favourite book and burned the silvery pockets of safety. With clear intent, he picked up the sewing scissors and held them to Jill's throat and raped her.

Jack hated Jill and for taking the pill
For he still wanted a daughter
He'd rape her here
And rape her there
And a pregnancy came following after

GOLDEN-EGG-THREE-BABY-BOY was born, having wrung sickness from his poor frail mother throughout his nine-month internment. Jill went back to work and every day, on her return, Jack would hold out his hand to take her wages from her to add to the sack of gold, which she never saw again. The squirrels watched from the high oak trees as Jill scuttled home each day, head down, beetling to avoid distraction, so she didn't miss her allotted-lift-time-slot back home to her Golden Eggs. The squirrels knew about hoarding, they knew how important it was to have a secret store of nuts, which no one else knows about, so when the hard times come, you can look after yourself and your own. They saw Jill hand over her money to Jack every twilight, before he would summon the lift and let her up so they knew Jack was looking after his own nuts and taking Jill's.

One night at the squirrel scurry, one huge, grey sow-squirrel squeaked out:

I'm worried about our neighbour Jill
She looks so tired and unhappy
Jack takes her cash
And don't give it back
Jill's trapped and beaten and battered

Her husband, a very kind old boar-squirrel concurred;

"I call on you today, mighty squirrel dray of Wide Oak Wood. My wife speaks the truth, for we have been watching with alarm as this poor human is daily bundled into the monstrous, alien, beanstalk, only returning to the forest floor at dawn."

"We have waited to see what the other humans will do, but poor pathetic species just turn their heads and shrug, giving away their power and claiming they can do nothing. Some even pretend blindness and deafness in order not to know what we squirrels know; that this stalk, is a stalk of suffering.

"We are small, but we are many and mighty and we know how to squirrel and hoard for harsh-iced-nights and frost-numbed-days and so we must do what we can to help Jill and her brood."

A cheer went up from the squiggling scurry and tiny, grey paws clapped in pride at the wise squirrel's call. As the dray quietened, the motherly-sow-squirrel spoke; "I will scamper with the human known as Jill as she makes her way through our paths and tracks to work tomorrow. I will whisper this plan to her in the human words I have been learning from YouTube. I will tell her that we The Wide-Oak-Wood Squirrel Dray will hoard her coins for her, keeping them safe in nooks and crannies so that when the ice comes and the snow falls, she has a store for herself and her chicks."

And so it was. Every day on the way home from work, Jill would drop a golden coin here and another there, so few that Jack didn't notice.

Every day the squirrels of Wide Oak Wood would scurry behind her, collecting the coins and caching them under muddy stones, within rotten bark, in mossy pillows and in tufted grass. Jill would watch their brushy tails, curling and furling and thank them with all her might.

Jack and Jill lived all alone
And Jill was really trapped here
She needed cash
To find her own home
So she and the kids could escape there

The three Golden-egg-boys grew into mighty fine chicks and Jill loved them with all her heart. She didn't care when the East wind blew in whispers that Jack was having an affair with a bra from the pub; it was just one less chore for her to do. Bra was welcome to him.

Golden-Chick-three was a sickly boy, who cried and cried and didn't like to sleep and Jill was exhausted; not sleeping, working, up and down the beanstalk all day long, just trying to keep on top of the housework while Jack drank and seduced in the bars and brothels of the wood.

O NCE UPON A TIME Jill was so, so tired from Chick-three's crying that her head was nodding over his pram. "I'll take care of him. Why don't you go for a sleep?" said Jack.

Hardly believing her ears, Jill gratefully turned towards her straw-mattressed pallet in the corner.

"Don't you walk away from me you witch" barked Jack.

Jill turned in time to see Jack launch the chick-filled-buggy, with one huge shove, so hard that it smashed and crashed against the farthest wall.

"That will shut him up" gnashed Jack before heading towards the lift and out again.

Jill didn't sleep then.

She knew she had to go.

In his haste, Jack had forgotten to deactivate the lift, now was her chance. She wrapped up her frightened golden chicks. She papoosed the still-breast-feeding-infant-three across her chest, funnelled the only-

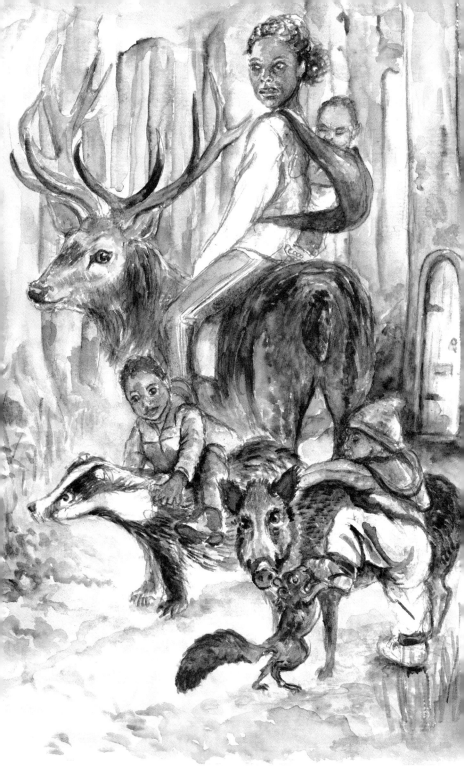

just-cruising-golden-chick-two into her baby backpack and took wobbly-walking-golden-chick-one's trembling hand in hers and safely descended the stalk; heart pounding, stomach churning, nose sniffing for Jack's return.

The squirrels of Wide Oak Wood had heard the affray, they had seen Jack stalk out, they had seen the door left uncommonly ajar and they sent whispers widely through the woods, that Jill needed the wood-folk's aid.

Emerging into the flora-green mist Jill gasped in amazement to find deer, rabbits, badgers and all the four-legged creatures of the woodland-kin-and-clan awaiting to bear her brood and she safely hence. Golden-chick-two wiggled and tiggled to get out and was excited to allow the neat pin-striped badger to snuffle him onto his back. Wobbly-walker-boy was greeted by the very calm, misunderstood, wild boar and the squirrels gave him a leg up for a ride. The proud red stag bowed his antlers that Jill may hold them to pull herself onto his soft, warm back, with her papoosed-still-infant-chick safe in her breast.

And so it was that Jill escaped the stalk.

The woodland creatures carried Jill and her brood to the edge of the wood, where they watched her swish and swash through the meadow grass, following the twinkling-star-nightlights to where her parents lay in their cool, crisp, unsuspecting bed.

Happy ever after.

The end.

E XCEPT BY NOW, you know it wasn't. It wasn't Happy Ever After nor was it the end.

Jill's parents sheltered the escaping brood until the nice people in the council gave them a home of their own. Houses in the meadow were too expensive by far, so Jill found herself back in the wood, but this time a little less afraid and a little more savvy.

The squirrels coin by coin, nugget by nugget, returned Jill's trove to her. She greeted their kindness with nuts from the chicks' outstretched palms and tears in her grateful eyes. She could do this, she could start a new life and not just survive, but thrive.

The squirrels told Jill that without her earnings, Jack's beanstalk had started to wither and die and that he was now living in a small hut, in the dark centre of the woods and was oft to be found carousing and brawling in The Dirty Dozen, The Thieves Lair or The Strumpet's Trumpet.

She had left with nothing and so lost everything, the little she had; her home-spun clothes, the babies' first rompers, shoes, coats, bags, the lot; all fell into Jack's hands, who sold them when he needed more ale.

Jack and Jill shared children still
So when he came to visit
He would steal Jill's purse
The chick's shoes and worse
So Jill looked like a bad mother

Because if Jack could make Jill look like a mad and bad mother, he could have the children taken away. Not that he wanted them, but he didn't want her to have them more.

Jill had made friends in the Wide Oak Wood and was invited out dancing with them. Jack, having promised to have the chicks that night, changed his mind last minute so her faithful and loving parents stepped in and wrapped them up snuggly and warm in the meadow nursery.

Off Jill went, bouncing happily along the woodland paths, happy to be free and with friends. She whirled and swirled and moshed and pogoed her way around the dance floor, laughing and sweating, hoping and releasing all the tension, the pain and the fear until, whoosh, she span into stalking Jack.

Push.

Shove.

Insult.

Accusation.

Slap.

At last the bouncers saw and threw him out, seething.

Jill carried on dancing.

As the stars started to fade and the blackbirds started to call to the chaffinch and the robin that dawn was approaching, Jill and her friend little Miss Muffet travelled home by stag, to Jill's new home, in Ash Tree Row.

"Be wary my ladies," warned the stag, "I think I saw someone moving in your house."

Jill knew it couldn't be, she had armoured glass and prison locks to keep her safe and sound.

Jill turned the many keys, in her many locks, and she and Miss Muffet stepped inside. Nothing in the hall. Nothing in the front room. A cold wind coming from the kitchen at the back of the house. Hearts beating, necks tensing, the girls pushed open the door to find shards of no-longer-armoured glass, slick with blood, scattered over the lino floor.

The police were called and this time came: policy had changed over the years, so now they did care about domestics, especially bloodied ones like these. They searched the house; following the blood trails up the stairs and pooling below the gaping, black wound of the loft-hatch-open. Jack was handcuffed, cursing, his glass-ripped arms and hands oozing venom and spleen.

"Love," said a departing officer, "hide the knife block in case he gets in again. You don't want to make it easy for him do you?"

Jack hated Jill and wanted to kill
So she took out a prohibitive steps order
Which kept him at bay
50 yards away
If he broke it the cops could take him away

ONCE UPON A TIME Jack slashed Jill's car tyres.

Once upon a time Jill found out that Jack's tragic-great-love fiancé who had died on the eve of their wedding, was in fact alive and had merely come to her senses and escaped when she could.

Once upon a time Jack called Jill to say "I'm coming to take the children away" and he called her from every phone box across the wood so she knew he was getting closer and closer. She called the police who came and took him away.

Once upon a time Jack told all the neighbours that Jill was having an affair.

Once upon a time, Jack came into Jill's house to pick up the chicks. When chick two said something Jack didn't like, Jack pinned him to the wall by this throat.

Once upon a time, chick two cut himself opening an ice cream and at the infirmary, Jack screamed and shouted at her for being an unfit mother, for being mad, for being bad, for being a screw-up, for causing her children harm.

Often upon many a time Jack threatened to take the children away.

Relentlessly upon a time Jack would threaten to kill Jill.

Eventually upon a time the police, having changed their attitudes to domestic abuse, took it in their own hands to prosecute Jack to keep Jill and the chicks safe.

The excess of fear she had felt in the stalk had inoculated her against his viral threats, life carried on. They were not out of the woods.

Her chicks grew and started to show the wounds of their childhood. Chick number one would cower at any sharp movement from where Jack had been batting him around the temples. He would sleep with the covers over his head and his fingers pressed in his ears from the rows he had heard, he would later need counselling for his anxiety and depression. Chick two didn't communicate or connect in the same way the other kids did and Jack told chick two he wished he'd never been born. Jack had chip, chip, chipped away at their happiness and safety. The guilt took hold of Jill and grew with every tremor, every shake, every withdrawal her children made; she had stayed too long. But how could she have got away sooner?

The woodland bramble network brought news that Jack had met another Jill, and that she too had planted the five beans, and was now living in Jack's new stalk, deep in the dark wood centre. Jack continued to drink and to batter, but still the courts said that chicks one, two and three needed to visit him. Jill-Too did her best to keep them safe and Jill one could do nothing but watch them go.

And then something happened which started to change Jack; his best friend 'accidentally' went too far one night when beating up his wife, and killed her. Oops. "It could have been me" the Jills told him. Shocked, at last into introspection, Jack stopped drinking and went to counselling. He tried to rebuild bridges with chicks one, two and three.

AND THEN JILL met Richard Whittington, who lived in the meadow, and knew the streets weren't paved with gold, so worked hard to make his own.

Rich and Jill met out with friends
Whilst Jill was finding her freedom
He drank coke
And could tell a joke
And didn't mind that she had children

He'd never once been in court
Could cook, wash and look after
She took him home
And made him her own
And lived happily ever after

And they really did.

In a small cottage, where the wood meets the meadow because now Jill is scared of neither and has a map and a compass to navigate both.

Happily married to this day.

They never row, they can talk about things.

Jack behaves himself now Richard is around.

Richard understands that she can't sit with him while he's watching the footy as his excited shouting flips her back into a fearful place, where she freezes and cowers and expects the worse.

Jill works with families, keeping kids safe, speaking out ever more strongly and clearly about abuse.

There can be happy enough endings in spite of the scars.

The chicks see their dad, and know he was bad
They are not deluded by daydreams
They can be in his home
But will leave him alone
When he starts to behave badly

Jack and Jill went up the hill
To fetch a pail of water
Jack fell down
And broke his crown
And Jill built a new life with another

Into the Woods

LIFE CARRIED ON.

Goldilocks found she loved teaching, found friends in her colleagues, occasionally flew back to visit Janine and ran, and ran, along tracks and sand, to keep the bears in her head at bay. She went on courses, read books and tried to understand what had happened to her, tried to make sense of it all.

Rapunzel, too, made a life for her children, found work and started to explore; what was it about her that had led her into not just one abusive relationship, but two?

Our beautiful Swan honoured her dream and went back to her studies and the dusty shelves of well-worn books. She found a group of women who helped her turn within and try to stitch the patchwork of her life together in a new quilt, in a pattern that made sense of the past and made the future warmer.

Sleeping Beauty's company thrives; she is respected and much loved.

Beauty Jane went back to school and learned all she could, so no other child would ever live through a life like hers on her watch.

Jill, too, made wisdom of her life and made it her business to protect children where she could, and to watch her own grow and make their ways into the world.

Naiad swam in the river, conserved her environment and raised her daughter to be at home in herself and in any element or weather, water or land, sun or rain, by rock or wave, in forest or meadow.

One day, sitting by the running river, Naiad wondered once again at the river's might. She knew where it started, just a small trickle high up in the heathered hills, and yet here, by her dew-wet fins, there was water enough for the ducks to play and the fishermen to cast, littering the banks with their pods of green and their flasks of steaming soup. She knew too that the river went on to join another a few miles hence, when, in heavy rain, it could halt the shoppers and the drivers, stop the familiar routes to school. Not content with their conjoined strength, the rivers did what all rivers do; headed to greater power, to greater velocity, to greater unity; to the sea. 'I wish', thought Naiad, 'that there were other women I could talk to, other women like me, who have been into the tall concrete prisons, the troubled waters and the dark forests. I wish I were not so alone with this story of mine'.

So when she saw the postcard in the window where the incense burned, calling her into the woods, she went.

Nervously. Without telling anyone.

She tucked her daughter into her walnut nest, in the sturdy wooden hut, by the snoozing stream, watched over by the wise owl and the alert vixen.

THE DUSKY PURPLING sky welcomed her wood-ward, and the first star winked in promise of what she was to find. The squirrels of Broad Oak Wood were tucking up their young and reading bedtime stories of scary humans and magical moons and the badgers were priming their noses for slug hunting and sharpening their ears to keep well away from the heavy, clumsy human feet. Heart beating, hat pulled down around her ears and cornflower hair, hands jammed in tissued pockets, fins snuggled in wool wraps against the cold and snags, she followed the breadcrumbs she knew not where. Until slowly, in the distance, she saw gloaming, a circle of golden, dancing flames of light beckoning her.

Stepping from the path into the tree-guarded circle she saw the faces turn to greet her and a crone, all dressed in midnight sky, reached out her gnarled hand to draw her into a wood-smoked embrace and onto a rug on the floor.

And so it was that our heroines met, protected by the canopy of stars and boughs. The oak offered its power and courage, the beech, its endurance and tolerance. The silver birch offered them new beginnings and the elm its intuition and inner strength. The ash brought its sensitivity, and the old witch hazel shared her wisdom and cleansing powers. The Sorceress-crone wove her way between the trunks, muttering and incanting, banishing Time from his busy distractions and closing the way to prying eyes.

The women watched as the cauldron bubbled on tripod feet over the flames, each wanting to run, wanting to stay, wanting to speak and then not knowing what to say or what had brought them to this wild spot on this still night in these broad woods. The Sorceress broke the silence, introducing the herbs as she sprinkled them onto the flames.

"Rosemary for remembrance, sage for wisdom, calendula for healing, chamomile for comfort, lavender for tranquillity, lovage for strength, thyme for courage, yarrow for healing and parsley for gratitude." The intoxicating scents filled the women's lungs and hearts and they settled more deeply onto Mother Earth who reassured them that she would hold them, no matter what, would keep them grounded and safe.

NVITING THEM TO stand, the Sorceress spoke; calling to the four directions to ask for their guidance. She called to the East for its qualities of air and clear communication, for new beginnings and new growth. She called to the South asking for its fire, its energy, its passion and creativity. She called on the West to share its power of water and emotion, of intuition and movement and she called to the North to bring its earthy qualities of security and home. Passing round a shell smouldering with dried herbs, she introduced the mugwort and directed the standing women to wash themselves in its smoke, cleansing away the detritus of their busy days and inviting them to turn inwards to their own truths, their own voices and their own hearts.

"Mother Earth, Father Sky, Grandfathers, Grandmothers, creatures of land, water and air we call on you to protect us here as we share ourselves tonight" intoned the Sorceress. "Guide us, teach us, protect and lead us in the direction of our highest purpose and our highest good that we may be sources for love and light in the world." She directed the women to sit as her ethereal ululations summoned the spirits of the twilit forest to their circle, the voices of women from far-off lands and from the dead and distant past until at last she sat and the circle was silent.

"Seek out a stone," commanded the Sorceress, "and bring it back to the circle." Each woman went their way, hugging their coats around them, cold away from the flames, strangers to each other still. They searched in tree roots, under mossy tree rot and leaf piles until each of them returned, holding their find tightly in nervous, muddied hands.

"It is now your time to speak" declared the Sorceress. "As we circle to your turn, speak your given name and then share what you will of your story that you may set yourself free from its hold. When you have said all your heart has to release, drop your stone into the cauldron and return to your place in the circle. If it is not your turn to tell your tale, you are a listener in silence. You have no more right to comment or question another woman's tale than you have the right to walk in her place to her home."

And so it began.

One by one the women shared their names and told their stories. The stars honoured their gathering and the moon waxed pregnant at what would be born from the tellings. The trees joined boughs in communion, keeping the space safe for the women and Mother Earth was nourished with their tears, supporting them, and welcoming them back into their own bones. The fire was fuelled by their suffering, their pain and their fears, leaping to consume each shred of self-doubt, shame and guilt and the air breathed its way deeply into their blood, clotting the wounds.

By the time the stories came to an end, the badger had eaten its fill and was curled up in its sett. The tawny sallied forth on midnight wings and the moths dithered around the fire from a safe distance. Silence once more settled like a blanket over the emptied women. Breathing in. Breathing out. The moment curled up around their shoulders and fell wordlessly asleep.

The Sorceress rose from her coal black cloak and shook her wild, silvered hair. Gesturing that they rise and join her, she started to disrobe and dance. Slowly, uncertainly at first, coats fell and socks wormed groundward. Soon shirts and dresses whirled their way in merry dances as the giggles and hoots held them in the air. As the fabrics dissolved, timeless figures formed. Sirens, Amazons and Goddesses took their places in the dance. Kali, Durga, Artemis, Athena, Hathor, Sekhmet,

Cleopatra and Boadicea swayed and swirled dervish-like in the reddish flames, chanting and howling to the wilds. Arms, legs, breasts, legs, thighs, living, dead, old, young, blurring boundaries, vibrating the air, tremoring the earth with their substance. Offering their blood, their stories, their lives, their souls to the circle, to each other, to women beyond the fire, beyond the wood, beyond their worlds.

Frenzied, the fire rose higher with each whoop and cackle, with each roar and shriek. The flames framed the faces of those who danced timelessly, endlessly, courageously to give birth to the new. Sweat mixed with tears, mud-coated feet and fins, blood-slimed thighs, hands reached for hands across the deserts of time and space to pull the women closer and closer still, until it seemed that the many had become one swirling, ageless woman, holding the whole of creation in her outstretched arms.

"We are enough!" thundered the Sorceress across the melee of gyrating flesh, and with a wave of her wand the fire flashed and returned to its stones and the women to their clothes. With another swoosh, the wand closed their eyes and lay them down, hand in hand, head in lap, arms slung across legs, soothing them to slumber and covering them with gossamer dreams.

O N AWAKENING, the Sorceress greeted them with a warming broth, of flavours so piquant and sublime that faces pinked and cells shook and stretched to welcome its nurturing home. "It is time," intoned the Sorceress, indicating to the women. "Reach into the cauldron and reclaim your stones.

"Eyes widened in fear at the gaping, steaming mouth of the boiling cauldron. How could they put their frail flesh in such torturous liquor and yet how could they not? It was Goldilocks who stepped forth, laughing bitterly that she'd faced pain before and would fear it no more. Silence waited for the scream and yet none came. Breaths released and eyes pierced the dancing shadows to see a small, white, unharmed hand clutching a chestnut-blooded stone. "I am Garnet, I give you self-worth and healing," announced the stone, widening eyes in the sistered circle.

Excited now, Beauty Jane peeped and peered but could not see

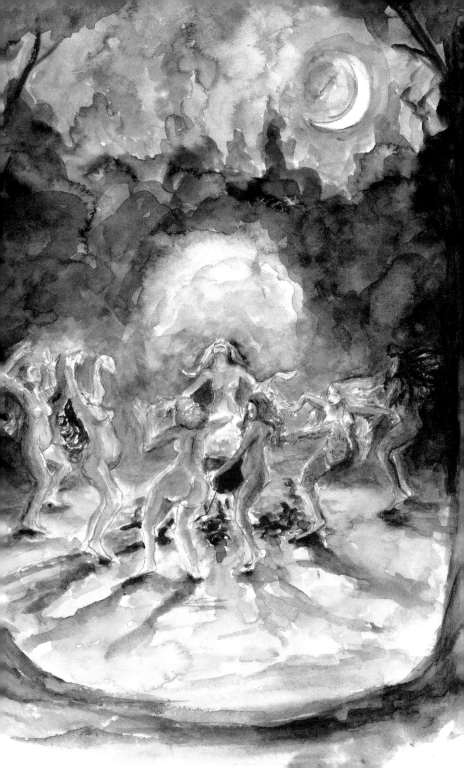

through the steam, so reaching in blind, birthed her rainbow stone of peony and gorse, which trilled its welcome to the awaiting crowd; "I am Tourmaline I give you joy and healing." Our Swan approached, pushing her feathered cloak clear and reaching in to find her grey, drab stone leap into her hand, transformed into a seascaped aquamarine blessing her with peace and clarity of communication. Rapunzel's undulating waves of emerald-mossy green proclaimed itself Malachite, keeper of protection and leadership.

Sleeping Beauty reached for Rose Quartz which blushingly blessed her with love and trust and Jill's shaking hand found a sunset Carnelian imbuing her with vitality and confidence. Naiad reached in at last to find sunrises in a stone; "I am Citrine," it giggled "I bring you clarity and imagination."

The peace was embroidered with the whispered confidences shared between the circle-sisters and their stones. Chuckling, calming, energising and empowering the aeon-old-earth-grandmothers shared their knowing and their power through the sinews and the neurons of their daughters, washing through bloodstreams with their offerings, delighted to be of service and in holds so dear and firm.

"You have told your tales and set yourselves free, you have danced with womenkind across time, you have found your own power and wisdom," said the Sorceress; "now it is time to share your knowing." She called them back to each other and watched as they bedded their stones, gratefully and warmly in gentle, plumped-up places.

"You have questions. Now is your time to ask, for each of you holds the wisdom each other needs" said the Sorceress to the moonish faces. They could hardly believe this to be true, but having seen base rocks turn into jewels and danced holding hands with deities, they inhaled, exhaled and dared to show what they didn't know.

"WHY DID THEY DO IT?" asked Rapunzel, "Why did both men I made children with treat me like a slave?"

"Because of their mothers" answered Beauty Jane.

"My man was beaten and shut up by his mother when he was young and scared and to hate her was just impossible, too scary, too dangerous so he pushed it down and packed it away and then when he met me, he took it all out on me. All that hate and violence he felt for her, he battered and inflicted into me, so I could feel as small and scared as he and so he didn't have to."

"I think it was because of his family" said Rapunzel. "They treated him like a God when he was growing up, he was the wage earner, the hero, even his mother and father did what he told them, so powerful was he in the home. He came from a family where the man is the boss, and so he was with me, he wanted to be in control of my every move. Both of them did."

"Because he was jealous," said Sleeping Beauty; "It only got really bad when I had my first child, he didn't like not being number one."

"Because of trauma" said Jill. "His dad died suddenly and he thought it was his fault. He never got over it."

"Because he was a narcissist" said Naiad; "He had a hole in his soul which wasn't filled when he was young and so everything was about him. He was incapable of empathy, or real love and care, because other people were only of interest if they were of use to him. Even our daughter."

"Because of the stories our culture tells us about men being strong, and dark and brooding" said the Swan. "Because we want someone dangerous to seduce and charm us and sweep us off our feet and take care of us. Because we have believed the films and books and tales which tell us that women secretly like to be dominated."

"Because they can," said the Beauty Jane. "Because the laws have let them for years and years, have let men own property, own the right to inherit, the right to vote, own women, rape their wives and bully and coerce without fear of punishment. These attitudes still run deep."

The women considered these answers and each found what they needed to be found.

"**D**O YOU THINK OUR childhoods made a difference?" asked Swan.

"I think so," said Goldilocks. "My mother was abused. I was abused as a child. My husband abused me much less. How could I know any different? I don't know what a healthy relationship with a man looked like. I'll never trust myself in a relationship again."

"I was brought up to be big and brave and strong and to never show any feelings, to lock emotions up and hide away the key, which meant I didn't feel fear or foreboding until it was too late" said Swan. "My parents were so critical, everything had to be perfect, nothing I ever did was good enough which was exactly how he treated me."

"It was my dad" said Naiad. "For so many years I wanted him to love and feel proud of me, but he was always so distant, so engaged in the outer world, he didn't have time for me. Only recently has he told me he is proud of me. All those years I never felt I was good enough, that I didn't please him, that he always thought I was wrong because I wasn't full mer or full naiad, I somehow didn't fit in with what I thought he wanted of me."

"I had to become a second mother," said Rapunzel; "And be a good Catholic Girl too of course; looking after the lads so they could go out and play."

"My father hit me," said Beauty Jane quietly. "And he used to look at me sexually when I hit puberty. I couldn't wait to leave home. From the frying pan into the fire."

"But mine weren't like that at all," said Sleeping Beauty; "the opposite in fact. They were so in love with each other and with us kids that we just didn't know how to spot bad people because we had never met any. We were so shielded and protected and their marriage was so romantic that we thought that was all there was."

"Mine are still like that. They've been together for ever" said Jill. "We were brought up to find peace and love in everyone. Maybe my father's childhood church would have served me better, maybe taught me how to spot a sinner."

"So we either went for men like our distant or critical or abusive parents or we didn't know how to spot a bad one because we'd been so wrapped up in cotton wool and blinded by Happy Ever After" said Naiad.

"So it would seem. But surely all that childhood stuff is still not enough to explain how I got hooked in?" said Swan;

"**H**OW DID I ALLOW myself to be reeled in and caught?"

"I fell for his charm," said Goldilocks; "He was so self-assured, he seemed so at ease, so in control, so relaxed, and he had money and good looks."

"He was so romantic" said Naiad. "He was so full of endearments and promises and whispers in ears and sensual sighs and strokes. He groomed me, he flooded me in words of love and I drowned in them."

"All the girls fancied him," said Beauty Jane; "He was a catch."

"The sex was amazing."

"I thought I could save him"

"Yes, somehow make him better, fix him, mend him"

"He was so charming."

"Yes so charming."

"I'd only met nice people" said Jill, "I had no idea that there were people in the world like him."

"Nor me" said Sleeping Beauty, "I had no discernment, no radar for darkness.""I was vulnerable" said Rapunzel; "I was a struggling single mother and he offered a home for me and my kids."

"I was naive."

"I was too trusting."

"I didn't listen to my intuition. Deep down inside I know that it felt wrong."

"I too was vulnerable" admitted Naiad. "My mum had just died and I was yearning to fill the hole in my belonging. I wanted a family of my own to fill the space my mother had been. And I was getting older, I thought it was the right time. Also I was alone in on a foreign shore, literally a fish out of water and I forgot to bring my compass, I had switched my internal bearings off."

"Me too" said Goldilocks; "I just wanted to be away from home, away from my father and brother, away anywhere seemed better. I didn't know him at all really."

"Me neither, not at all" said Naiad.

"I wasn't in a strange land, but I isolated myself" said Jill. "I stopped seeing people, I stopped going out, I stopped telling the truth so in the end it was just me and him."

"So charm, then isolate?" asked Swan.

"Then harm" sighed Beauty Jane. "Once there was no one for me to turn to for help, it got bad."

"When I had kids" said Jill.

"Me too" said Sleeping Beauty.

"Charm, isolate, harm" said Swan; "Systematic and simple but invisible until it's too late."

"WHAT I DON'T understand" said Rapunzel, "Is why I didn't get out at the first sign."

"Because it's incremental" said Naiad; "It starts small, and you let it go, ignore it, delete it, pretend it's OK, explain it away, but it's growing and growing."

"Because we were brought up to believe that marriage needs work and so I worked at putting up with it," said Jill.

"Also, they're not bad all the time" said Goldilocks. "To start with he was so kind, so gentle and he could be every now and then. The promises of how good life together would be was so convincing."

"If only I was a little bit better, sexier, more loving, different, then things would be OK, so you keep on trying to change yourself to make him happy and you get so worn down with his constant criticisms that you begin to believe that it is all your fault" said Swan.

"Because we've been brought up to believe that love will conquer all, that love will heal, that we have to stand by our man, for better for worse, for richer, for poorer," said Sleeping Beauty.

"I remember my teenage magazine, all about how to meet your perfect boy," said Beauty Jane.

"All those love songs, all that romance," said Jill.

"And the stories," said Sleeping Beauty. "I was a sucker for Mr Rochester and Heathcliff; wounded passion to be cured by the love of a good woman."

"Me too," said Naiad.

And don't forget the films we grew up with, where the man always came to the rescue, all big and strong," added Rapunzel.

"We were brainwashed," said Jill.

"We were," they all agreed.

"**B**UT WHY DO we put up with that?" asked Naiad; "None of us are stupid."

"I was brought up to please people, to look after the men and so I just carried on doing that" said Rapunzel.

"Me too," said Beauty Jane. "I was scared of my father so it just felt normal to be scared of him."

"Same for me," said Goldilocks, "Fear is so normal".

"I've learned I'm co-dependent," said Rapunzel.

"What's that?" asked Jill.

"It's when you only feel good when you are making other people happy and so you never do anything to make yourself happy. In fact you don't really have a sense of self outside of other people, you only exist to serve and please others. I learned as a child; keep the peace, be a good girl, please others and do as you're told."

"I was so obedient," said Swan. "I think it's because in school if you didn't do what you were told, you got into trouble and I always did what I was told at home too."

"I think that's true," said Rapunzel; "I had home and school and the church; I was going to Hell if I didn't do what I was told, so I just did what I was told with men too."

"I was going to Hell too, my father assured me of that and my husband made that threat come true." said Beauty Jane; "But for me the obedience wasn't incremental, it was sudden, the moment he put his hand through the door, my mind went blank and I did what I was told."

"Terrifying" said Swan.

"I think it was stress" said Goldilocks; "I was so shocked and scared the first time my father did something bad to my mother in front of me that my mind shut down and I couldn't think straight and so when my father did that to me, he already had control. So no wonder I just gave up my life to my husband and his family. I still have flashbacks and nightmares about it all. I'm always feeling scared and on the lookout for threats.

"No matter what I do, how much I learn, where I go, how much I run, I can never sit still. My solar plexus is always as tight as a drum, my heart pounds at the slightest thing. I don't trust myself let alone men. I'm always alert for danger, wired for threat, expecting the worst.

"I'm waiting for some new treatment, something called EMDR. I've no idea how it works but apparently it takes the power from the memories, takes the pain away. I can't imagine it will. I don't even know if I can face telling my story to a stranger. Although", she smiled at the eyes holding her eyes in their care, "I just have".

"I know those nightmares too," said Sleeping Beauty.

The trees drew a breath, the earth paused while the sadness settled and was absorbed.

"I had children," said Jill; "I'd been brought up to believe that children needed two parents, so I stayed."

"Me too, I just wanted to be a happy family and I tried and tried, for too long," said Sleeping Beauty.

"I thought I owed it to my daughter to stay married, so she knew her dad," said Naiad.

"But it's not just that is it? Not just us. It's what the media says about broken families and single mothers and the damage divorce does to kids and I didn't want that to happen to mine," said Beauty Jane angrily. "It's always the single mother who gets the blame. No one blames the man who left."

SILENCE FELL as they nodded their agreement.

"So many of you suffered physical violence," sighed Swan.

"Yes and it's always emotional and psychological too. Telling you you're a bad mother, calling you names, telling me he'd take the children away and threatening to hurt them too," said Jill. "And rape at knifepoint."

"Rape all the time," said Beauty Jane.

"Yes all the time," said Goldilocks. "With my father I had no choice, he was too strong and I was too young. With my husband, I didn't even know I had a right to say 'no'."

"He raped me to get me pregnant, because then I was more trapped," said Jill.

"He strangled me. I thought I would die," said Beauty Jane.

"Mine strangled me too," said Jill.

"I read it's quite common," said Goldilocks; "it leaves no marks and is hard to spot but can cause brain damage. My poor mum."

"I feel like a phony," said the Swan; "mine was only ever critical and mean, maybe I didn't experience actual abuse."

"Of course it was," said Naiad; "that stuff's illegal now; coercive control; persistent and systematic, controlling you by doing your head in."

"By promising to do something and then letting you down."

"By lying."

"By cheating."

"By moving your things around and denying it so you feel like you're going mad."

"By checking your phone and computer."

"By smashing things."

"By stalking you."

"By never helping with the house or kids."

" By telling you you're mad."

"By not letting you go out."

"Or saying you can go out but then creating a row so you are too upset to go."

"Or by making you feel so ashamed that you don't want to go."

"Or by insulting your friends so they drift away."

"Or frowning and growling when they come round, so they don't come around any more."

"He turned the kids against me."

"He told mine lies."

"He turned mine against each other."

"He threatened to take me to court."

"To take them away."

"So I'd never see them again."

"I was so ashamed, so full of shame at what he did. I believed him when he said it was all my fault" said Beauty Jane.

"So ashamed."

"And scared too," said Jill.

"I was scared."

"I was scared."

"Me too."

"Me too."

"Mine controlled me through money," said Rapunzel; "He kept me poor."

"So you couldn't leave. I know that too. I had to squirrel money away, a pound here and a fiver there, it all took so much time," said Jill.

"Mine locked me in the house, or hid my key so I couldn't go out."

"Mine too. Locked me in or locked me out. Either way was bad."

Their hearts beat steadying their breath.

"DID ANYONE HELP you get out?" asked Swan; "I went to my sister who was a star."

"My mum came up trumps in the end and my brother too," said Beauty Jane.

"We went to family therapy but it didn't work," said Sleeping Beauty.

"Nor for us," said Beauty Jane.

"Because he didn't want to change, because it was never his fault," said Sleeping Beauty.

"The police were useless the first time," said Jill. "they sent me back home to sort it out and just didn't want to get involved."

"They put orders in place to keep him away," said Beauty Jane.

"Yes for me too. Eventually," said Goldilocks.

"I didn't know about the court orders until I was out and safe," said Beauty Jane. "My solicitor didn't understand domestic abuse even though she knew what was going on. So I missed out on protections we were due."

"Mine was good, they sorted him and the house," said Swan.

"I left him the house, even though it was mine," said Sleeping Beauty.

"Me too," said Jill.

"Me too," said Beauty Jane.

"I left with nothing," said Goldilocks.

"He went for everything," said Naiad.

"I just didn't have the energy to fight."

"The police did help in the end," said Jill; "times are changing."

"Not fast enough."

"WHAT MADE YOU leave in the end?" asked Swan. 'I was on holiday with him just before my 30th birthday when he hit me for not listening to him and I thought 'I'm not going to stay living like this when I'm 30'."

"He tried to hit my daughter, and then I had time off work with stress and the river lightholders came around and built my confidence bit by bit, until I felt strong enough to leave him," said Naiad.

"Work helped me," said Sleeping Beauty; "I went to a conference where we did an exercise that made me realise how I never looked after myself. I went home and ended it that night."

"There was no one thing, I just knew I had to go for my children's sake," said Rapunzel.

"I left after he slammed my baby's buggy across the room, into the wall, with my son in it," said Jill.

"I knew I had to go when he made me abort my only child. I had no choice, he drove me there and spoke for me and I was too scared and confused and didn't know what was happening or how I would manage as I had no money or home of my own. But when I saw myself there, on that bed, with the men with silver instruments between my legs and all the blood, I had a flashback to when I was young, when my father punched and kicked my mother until she bled and then I understood for the first time, in that moment, as my own child was dying, that my father had killed my brother or sister while still inside my mother's womb and I knew then, I had to get out. Had to find a way to escape. And I did. But it took years."

Heads bowed. Fingers wiped tears from eyes. Hands were held. Pause. Breathe. Continue.

"His mother came round to the house," said Beauty Jane, "accusing me of all kinds of things and I just lost it, and screamed at her listing all the things he'd done. Of course she wouldn't hear it of her darling son, but I knew I wasn't safe after that. I put the kids in the car and went to my brother's house."

Words stopped for thought. Hands reached to warm by the fire, legs stretched, blankets pulled closer, before leaning in for more.

"**D**ID HE STAY in touch afterwards?" asked Swan; "I only ever heard from him again when social media arrived and I blocked him."

"I wish it were that easy," said Naiad; "I have to have contact with him because of our daughter. He still uses her for control, often cancelling at the last minute and letting her down, we can never make any plans and he has never paid a penny. He lied in court about his cash-in-hand work; pleading poverty and all the while hiding stacks of cash under his bed, invisible."

"My kids are older now so they make their own arrangements," said Jill; "But to start with he would let down my tyres, make death threats, threats to take the kids. He broke into my house once, hid my things and got one of the kids by the throat. It went on for years. The courts were useless and he didn't ever give me any money for the kids."

"He had me by the throat after I left, with a knife, I was sure I would die" said Beauty Jane. "It was only when I met someone else that things calmed down; maybe that's why I married again, he kept me safe, and helped raise the boys."

"He threatened to kill himself too." said Jill.

"Mine too," said Sleeping Beauty; "but he loved himself too much to ever do it."

"So none of you have had a penny to raise the kids?" asked Swan, incredulous.

"Never."

"Never."

"No, nothing at all."

"Why not?" asked Swan.

"He hid it."

"He got paid in cash so it couldn't be tracked."

"I was too scared to ask."

"I didn't want him turning the children against me."

"The courts couldn't make him pay."

"I got sick of asking."

"So how did you manage?" asked Swan.

"Worked."

"Worked."

"Worked."

"Worked and did it all myself."

"Yes kids, work and home."

"Yes, I do it all, it's exhausting."

"Then my new partner helped."

"Mine too."

"Do you think it harmed your children?" asked Swan, whose children had come to her after she escaped, when she was safe, when she had built a new home.

And now the tears came apace, the arms went round shoulders that heaved and heads that bowed. The moon watched steadily and the trees drew in closer to keep them safe as they wept for the children, their unborn children, their children who had deserved better, deserved more and didn't get it. Shame shrouding the mothers, pointing out how they had failed to protect their most beloved, how they had left it too long. The tears wet the earth who accepted them home and seeded their hopes for a better future for them all.

"Mine developed asthma that cleared once we were free."

"Mine suffers from depression."

"Mine sees a counsellor and still can't put it all to rest."

"Mine has low self-esteem and is in an abusive relationship herself."

"Mine has difficulties building relationships in school."

"Mine won't talk about it. They were silenced by it."

"I will never have a child. He killed my only one"

The leaves stilled, the beetles ceased their scurrying, the Sorceress bowed her head and Time stretched his unused limbs and went back to sleep.

A slow moaning Om trailed across the flames, drawing the women in. They added their voices one by one, keening, wailing, swaying, clinging, sobbing, retching. The sharp notes soared skyward, star-ward, reaching to be transformed and healed. But there was no healing. Some scars just have to be borne. Some holes can never be filled and the suffering of a child should never be stilled. The lamentation slowly settled into their hearts, mingling with melancholia, searching for acceptance but finding none. It hushed slowly in the rocking arms of loving mothers who had done their best but failed to keep their children safe from harm.

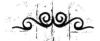

"THERE IS ONE more question" said the Sorceress; "What did you learn?"

"Nothing," said Swan. "I wish I'd never met him. I wish I hadn't stayed with him for so long. I wish I'd done what I wanted to do instead of worrying about him."

A pensive quiet was broken when Rapunzel spoke; "I learnt to look after myself and be financially secure, have a backup plan. I'd never move into someone's house until I've taken the time to get to know them – a long time. I'm learning how to be stronger now, to look after myself and care for myself. I know now that I'm as important as anyone else. When you love yourself you're less likely to put up with anyone else's shit. I've had to learn about my co-dependence and sort it out."

"I've had to learn to look after myself. I'm as hard as rock for myself, I can manage, it's the kids who make me cry," said Beauty Jane.

"I think it made me stronger. It made me more assertive. I think the repercussions of a broken relationship do just ripple on. I think it hardened me, it's probably seriously hardened me in personal relationships. I don't need anyone. I'm alright on my own. It is a disillusionment," said Sleeping Beauty. "I'm over-protective of my sons." She swallowed hard. "I needed an injection of; 'These are your rights and you matter and what you want matters.' What I probably needed were some different messages in early childhood."

"I wish I could tell my younger self to just walk away, tell someone, refuse to go home," said Goldilocks. "I should have made more of a fuss.

But times were different then. I didn't know there was help. I didn't think that anyone would believe me. I didn't think I was worth the fuss, worth saving. I never go out, I don't trust people. It took all my strength to come here tonight. I felt sick, I would have run away if there had been a man here. I have panic attacks. I can't imagine trusting another man ever. I never thought I would be able to sit in a circle and talk like this. I'm only here on a visit. My friend Janine persuaded me to come."

"It has made me stronger. Before I was the crusader and the fixer, always looking out for the underdog. I still want to fix things and people and solve problems but I'm getting better at thinking, 'It's not my problem' and walking away." said Jill. "It would have helped if people had talked about it more. No one talked about it; it was taboo. It didn't happen to people like me. I thought it was just me. Now I know it's not."

"I think I was a dreamer, I had heard too many stories and wanted romance and happy ever after. I missed my mum, I was lonely, I wanted kids and thought I needed to be married to do that. I didn't. I was so busy being a good woman, a good wife, that I didn't look after myself. I was so used to pleasing people and being a good girl. I had no boundaries." said Naiad. "I'd never felt hatred until I was getting away from him. I thought that nice girls don't have nasty feelings like hatred. Then I worked out that hatred is my emotions' way of making sure I don't get hurt again."

"I was the same. I grew up without healthy conflict. I had no idea of my rights. We were all nice people, people pleasers, I got all those lessons – 'Put other people's needs before your own' and 'Never stand up for yourself or look after yourself'. All that. Now I do." added Sleeping Beauty.

She continued; "I wish someone had said to me, 'Don't take anyone on potential. What you see is what you get'. If you've got a cat they're going to meow, if you've got a dog they're going to bark, if you've got someone who manipulates you they are going to keep manipulating you. Just see it and walk away. Know that you will be fine and that you are strong. Reach out for more support, tell more people, trust other people more, listen to what they say, don't make excuses, don't mistake pity or fixing for love. Put yourself right in the frame and ask yourself; 'What do I want from a relationship' not 'What do I need to give this person in order to make them happy'."

The women nodded in agreement and gazed once more into the flames, their stones nesting in closer as balm for their hurting hearts.

THE SORCERESS stood once more, holding her staff before her, her eyes fierce with love and protection, and spoke; "You have grown your courage by putting your hands in the cauldron and sharing your pains. You have grown your connection by moistening your sisters' skins with your tears. You have shrunk your shame by naming it. You have softened your hearts by declaring your losses. You have found your voices in your lamentations. You have regained adventure by following the breadcrumbs. You have gained wisdom by learning and joining the dots to make meaning. You have reclaimed your own story by creating these narratives. You have connected with nature by sweating into her arms. You have found your own wildness in your dervish swirling. You have seen your womanhood mirrored back through the aeons.

"You have gained much from each other and with each other tonight, but your work is not done. Look around you sisters, look with your skin and your bones, sense with your tongue and your touch, feel with your heart and your intuition, listen with the ears of a wolf, sniff, scrape, dig, test, taste, for each of you must find your spot in this circle, a spot of your own." With that she pulled her cloak around her and appeared to be laying down to sleep.

"What do you mean our spot?"

"How will we find it?"

"How will we know?"

"You will know," was the last thing the Sorceress would say before pulling her cloak over her silken, magnesium mane and resting her head on the mossy pillow to sleep.

At first, they chatted as they looked; gossip, families, work and the like. Laughing at this, the most prosaic and bizarre of tasks.

"Let's just sit somewhere and tell her we've found our spots."

"She'll know."

"That's cheating," they giggled.

Cold away from the fire, their voices stilled and their searching sharpened. Sifting leaf dust, untucking moss blankets, sitting here, leaning there, lying on their fronts then on their backs. Slowly deepening into their own searches. Sharp tangs, soft smudges, garlic, mould, bitter, tart, sharp, smooth, uneven, shadowed, ticking, a slight hiss. Feral, they dug deep, climbed high, inhaled the space with every pore and orifice, entranced. This spot colder, this darker, this light, this rippling, like currents in summer seas, unseen oscillations, vibrating through them, each one, together, yet alone. Hands and knees pawed, guts sensing, backs of necks quivering, ears pricking, tongues dripping, skin roughening, untamed, undomesticated, untrained they stalked their prey until tiring, silently, they fell to slumber one by one.

Waking to pipes playing, the women stretched their boughs and shed their blankets of leaves and bracken carefully placed for warming during their slumber. Smiling, the Sorceress bid them rest in their coverleted fronds saying; "My daughters, you have found your sweet spots and completed your final task."

Confused they protested:

"I was tired and fell asleep."

"I couldn't find it so I just slept here."

"There was nothing magical about it."

"Yes, just a normal spot to rest."

"Ah" replied the elder; "Why did you chose that spot to ease your weariness?"

"It felt comfortable."

"And warm."

"And safe."

"And solid."

"And soft."

"It sort of welcomed me."

"Yes, like it was pleased to see me."

"Just accepted me."

"Made space for me."

"Didn't cramp me."

"Didn't demand anything of me."

"I felt good there."

"Felt content."

"Felt easy."

"Felt like it just suited me without me having to try."

"I could breathe easy."

"And relax."

"I liked being there."

"I could be myself."

"I was happy to be there."

"I love this spot."

As they spoke, their smiles grew, their amusement bubbled, their wonder glowed and they knew that they had found that spot with their gut, with their heart, with their wildish, witching nature, their inner knowing, their intuition untrammelled or tamed by fairy stories and laws.

"Granddaughters," spoke the older woman, "remember this, for this is how love feels. It is like the earth constant beneath your feet, the sun warming you, the rivers quenching your thirst, the woods giving your shelter, the air urging you to fly. It has seasons and storms, it waxes and wanes, there is nothing but constant change; growth and decay and regrowth. And so it is with all things. And so it should be. And so it is. Remember this well."

"Your sweet spot of earth holds a gift for you. Reach into the mother's womb and ask her to birth it to you in remembrance of this time and space."

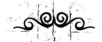

TRUSTING NOW, the women did as the crone instructed and tenderly, gently, sensitively, pushed their fingertips into the source of their growing, giving thanks for her holding, her resting place, her abundance, her diversity and her equanimity.

The loam crumbled under each tender touch, opening, elbow deep as each woman reached inside her own sweet spot to find what was held for her there.

"A golden heart," announced Naiad; "It's strange; soft yet strong, it gives and yet is firm, it's sweet, but can't be crushed" she observed. "Oh look! It opens! When I breathe on it, when I breathe slowly, when I'm calm," she exclaimed, amazed, looking inside to find two pictures; "My daughter and me. But it's not me now. It's me as I would like to be, healthy and happy and whole. The me that I really am." she declared as she gazed and turned her glowing heart for all to see.

"What's this?" said Sleeping Beauty perplexed, as she opened a cardboard box and pulled out a big black box, with ant-eyes grille and dials and knobs. "An amplifier!" she giggled, "It's what I needed in my marriage, I needed to listen to my own inner voice which knew things weren't right. I needed to speak my truth more loudly and clearly and look after myself more. So many of the women I work with today need one of these! I'll keep it in my office to remind us all that we have a voice and have a responsibility to make ourselves heard."

The moments paused mid-flight, hovering, delicately allowing the instant to expand and take root before Swan held her new-found looking glass by its pearly, slender neck, nonplussed. "A mirror," she announced flatly. She held it to her face and was met by her own sad eyes, her own lined skin, her greying hairline, her crinkling neck and she pulled it away abruptly, letting it hang limply by her side, disappointed.

"Look again" commanded the Sorceress, "But this time look with the eyes of love."

Slowly, begrudgingly, Swan obliged, turning her head away, disliking what she saw.

"What would love see?" asked the Sorceress.

"I don't know, I can only see..."

"Stop. Look as your daughters would see you, look with the eyes of your friends, with the soul of your husband and tell us what you see."

Slowly Swan saw. She saw the sad eyes of one who has survived what could not be escaped and who escaped when the time was right. She saw courage in the alert shoulders, the jutting chin. She saw laughter crowing around her eyes and she saw the wisdom and wit of her silvered hairs. She saw intelligence in the furrows on her brow and curiosity in her raised eyebrow. She saw a certain ironic smirk lingering in the corner of her mouth, and lips still plump for kissing. She saw strength in her cheekbones, kindness in her ruddied cheeks and when she looked deep into her own eyes, she felt waves of love and compassion for this woman who she was, who she had been and who she was becoming.

Beauty Jane held out the photograph of two smiling boys, tears dripping down her arm, pooling in the crook of her elbow before reaching down to the ground below. "My boys," she gulped and choked. "I love them so much my heart breaks at the hurt they have to live with."

"Who are they smiling at?" asked the Sorceress.

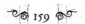

"Me. They are smiling at me" cried Jane Beauty. "They still always smile at me" she said smoothing their smiles with her shaking, dirtied fingers.

"Why do they smile at you?" asked the sorceress. "Remember."

"Because I make them smile, we have a laugh, we always did, even in the darkest hours. I would bite my hand so the children didn't hear my fear and pain, I would laugh it off to keep them safe. We would sing and play and dance when he was away and we would make dens for bear hunts and castles in the sand. When they were older I was there for sports days and homework and eventually girls. I've worked with them, I've lived with them as adults. We go on holidays, we talk, we share, we trust each other."

"So were you a good enough mother?"

"I hope I was."

"Yes you were. You are. You will always be. It wasn't your fault."

Rapunzel held a heavy, brass padlock with a polished golden key that released the arch to open and clicked assertively when shut. So weighty and solid, and cold to touch, she saw at once why it was hers. "This is perfect!" she laughed. "A lock reminds me of so many things. A room of my own so that I can lock myself away to do what pleases me and me alone. A lock to my own house, I'll never be co-dependent again. A lock to set boundaries, to say; 'No thank you, not today for I am busy looking after my own needs and making myself happy'. A lock to remind me that I am free and that the only person who can lock me in is me so let me out and throw away the key!"

The women's laughter subsided as they turned to Jill who was leaning against a solid oaken shield that reached from her feet to her hips and was twice her width. "I am this shield" said Jill. "I did what I was able to shield the children with my own life to keep them safe against knife or fist or throw. I shielded myself as best I could, saving money, staying sane and then escaping when I could. Now I'm safe I am the shield for other mothers in my work, I protect their children and help them escape. I teach people what I have learned, I speak out to shake things up faster and easier so that no one has to live like I did. Not on my watch. I am proud of this shield. I am proud of me."

Last of all they turned to Goldilocks holding a book. "I have read so much to try and understand what happened to me. I have studied and I have learned and I have turned within. I have written what I know to teach and share, to educate, to illustrate. I have written what I wish I had known. What I wish I had read before it was too late, before I was embroiled and stuck. I have written so that all can spot the signs and stay away or reach for help before it's too late. This book I hold now is blank. Its pages are fine and heavy, they smell fresh, they are empty. I want to write a different story now."

HE SORCERESS gathered them to the circle around the fire, where the cauldron still gurgled and steamed. As she waved her wand the flames quietened. She turned to Time still sleeping beyond the circle and whispered him awake. Time stretched the light into the distant dawn. The blackbird shook his feathers and heralded the morning and the robin hopped from branch to branch; "It's time to wake up, it's time to wake up".

Reaching into the cauldron she ladled its contents into the eight chalices at her feet. Taking one herself, she beckoned the women take their own.

"What is it?"

"It looks like water."

"It tastes like water."

"Was it water all along?"

"You are your own gifts, your own treasures, your own jewels. For magic is water, it flows through us all. It is common and plentiful once we understand that magic is the power that turns this wizened, dried, acorn into that bud and then that huge old tree and then back into the ground as mulch. Magic is the power of connection, of sharing, or reaching out to one another. You need nothing more than yourself."

"Go now into the world and share what you know with the women who are not here tonight, who can't escape, who are scared and tired and confused. Find those women and their children and talk to them. Share your stories. Nurture them. Help them. Be their safe place. What happens to one of us happens to us all. We are all just walking each other home."

As the sun rose the fire faded and the women took their leave. The trees stepped back into their places, their circle to be reconvened on another such night. The squirrels hurried their babies from sleeping dens and the wood-anemones held up their petals in delight. The Sorceress returned to her day-life, hair tucked neatly away behind her ears, cloak carried in a battered bag. Not even the fire embers remained.

The women had no need for breadcrumbs; for each now knew how to find her own way in and out of the woods.

As Naiad walked along her river towards her sturdy house where her child slept, she knew that she was a drop that would make up a trickle that would join with another to make up a stream, that would meander to join other rivers, expanding and making waves and turning tides in all the seas.

Seeing the Wood for the Trees

O, THERE WE HAVE THEM, the facts, the fictions, all mixed up; just like real life. While all of us got out of the woods alive, we are aware that not all do. None of us made it out of the woods without help, whether from real people, agencies or what we read and understood. Here are the things that helped us either by practically offering support or just by helping us understand and therefore forgive ourselves more and more. May they help you and yours.

DOMESTIC VIOLENCE HELPLINE UK freephone, 24 hours, confidential 0808 2000 247

BANDURA

Bandura was a psychologist who showed how we are influenced by people who are more powerful than us, the same gender as us and who we see often, which goes some way to explaining why we copy our same-sex parent.

Also Bandura helped me understand why we'd fallen for the whole romantic myth, shedding some light on why we fall for the myths of the Perfect Romance, Perfect Family, Perfect Prince and Princess; we are bombarded with these images and expectations in advertising and films, books, music and social media and these unrealistic ideals become the sticks we use to measure our lives against and beat ourselves with.

BOWLBY

Bowlby was a psychologist, psychiatrist and psychoanalyst well-known for his interest in child development and his work in attachment theory. He helped me understand how early childhood attachments can have an effect on later adult relationships, as relevant for the abuser as well as the abused.

BROWN
Brene Brown's Ted Talk is one of the most watched ever. She is a qualitative researcher who has studied, in depth, the nature of shame; what shames us and how shame affects us. She really helped me understand how shame had kept us locked in and shut off from help.

THE BYSTANDER EFFECT
Latané and Darley's research explains why so many people stand by and do nothing when they know that abuse of any kind is occurring. We all think that people will do something about it so we don't have to. Then no one does anything and the abuse is allowed to continue. It is now against the law not to take action when you are aware that a child is at risk of harm and as these stories show, children are harmed when there is domestic abuse. We all have to step up and take action when we think that abuse is occurring, it is all of our responsiblity.

LOCAL COUNCIL CHILD PROTECTION
If you are concerned about a child then these are the people to contact unless there is an immediate crisis in which case call the police. The Child Protection Team are really happy to talk about the legal process, CAFCASS and the ways that they assess harm.

CO-DEPENDENCE
Learning about co-dependence helped me to understand that this was the way that I made myself vulnerable to being abused. I was so eager to make him happy, to keep the peace, to meet everyone else's needs and to be the martyr to myself that I was the perfect fit for him. Coda run support groups and awareness training to help people stop being co-dependent which Rapunzel found really helpful.

CRAVEN
Pat Craven worked with abusers in prison and in so doing, came to understand the varying behaviours abusers use to gain control through sex, violence, money, isolation, intimidation, bullying, threatening and fucking with your mind. Her work is the basis of the Freedom Programme.

FREEDOM PROGRAMME

This is a confidential group course which is offered for free to bring victims together to learn about abuse and gain peer support; invaluable.

FREUD

Now I know Freud gets a bad rap for all his penis fascinations, but he also has some really helpful concepts. He was the first person to introduce the idea of 'defence mechanisms' which is what our conscious brain uses to protect itself from something that is too much to bear. Denial is when we don't want to see the truth of a situation and repression is when we push down our feelings as they aren't safe to express them and it certainly seemed from the interviews that these were part of why we stayed for so long. Projection and transference also helped Beauty Jane understand the Beast; he hated his mother but couldn't acknowledge those feelings, so transferred those feelings onto Jane.

LAW AND THE POSITION OF WOMEN IN SOCIETY

The law is a huge influence and indicator of gender roles and when I looked at the legal history between men and women it made shocking reading and helped me see how social rules and norms about the position of women have led to some of the attitudes that perpetuate abuse today.

It was only from 1870 that women could own their property, up until this time any property a woman had was transferred to their husband on marriage. In 1922 men and women had equal rights to inherit property. If you wanted to buy your own house, even in 1970, women couldn't get their own mortgage but had to have their husbands sign for them. Anita Roddick of Body Shop had to ask her husband to sign for her loan for her first shop as the bank wouldn't consider her. Only in 1980 could women apply for a loan or a credit card in their own names.

The Equal Pay Act only came into force in 1970 thereby making it illegal to pay women less than men. However, statistics still show that women still are paid less than men, are promoted less often and hold fewer board-level jobs even though there was an amendment in 1985 which allows women to be paid the same as men for work of the same value. In 1975 the Employment Protection Act made it illegal to sack a woman when she is pregnant. Up until this point, pregnant women were financially dependent on their partners or families so the possibility of surviving alone would have been nigh on impossible.

Only in 1956 was rape defined within the Sexual Offences Act, up until this time there was no such thing as the crime of rape and it was only in 1972 that Erin Pizzey set up the first women's refuge for victims of domestic abuse. Horrifically, it was only in 1995 that rape in marriage became illegal. It was 1997 before the register for sexual offenders was set up. Coercive control was recognised as a crime in late 2015 and police are now given more training in tackling domestic abuse. However, the office of national statistics found that 1.4 million women suffered domestic abuse last year.

Having a good solicitor who understands domestic abuse is critical so that Prohibitive Steps Orders and Restraining Orders can be used to keep victims safe.

Milgram

Stanley Milgram wanted to understand how perfectly nice Germans did what they did in World War Two and in so doing, taught the world about the way we become obedient. We become obedient to people who we perceive as having more power than us and this is more likely to happen when we are in close proximity to them, for example, living with them. The control is incremental, it creeps up on us so in the end we don't think for ourselves. This really helped me forgive myself for allowing the situation to develop as it did; I didn't notice the incremental control it until it was too late and by then I felt stuck.

Narcissistic Personality Disorder

So many of the abusers fit this profile; the inability to empathise, the need for constant attention and adoration, only doing things that make them look good, using other people for their own ends, arrogance, grandiosity, envious, controlling. Reading books about this was like someone putting the floodlights on. These people are charmers as long as they are getting what they want, they are skilled manipulators and as far as I know, cannot be cured, not least because, of course, they don't see that there is anything wrong with them, it is always everyone else's fault.

Police

Call 999 if you are in danger or 101 if you are worried about the threat of danger. Even if the police don't act, you have record of the abuse which can help in later court cases.

Post-Traumatic Stress Disorder

I used to think that only war veterans suffered from this, but it turns out that people living with abuse do too. It shuts off your ability to think straight and makes you hypervigilant, slow to trust and frightened long after the abuse has stopped. EMDR (Eye Movement Desensitization and Reprocessing) seems to be one of the most effective treatments for post-traumatic stress and can be obtained on the NHS as well as privately.

Skinner

Skinner was a psychologist whose work reveals how we are all controlled by positive and negative reinforcement or punishment. To get people to do what we want them to do we can either reward them when they do it, or punish them when they don't. The control, or conditioning, works best when the pattern of reward or punishment is unpredictable, it is, for example, why gamblers keep gambling. It is also why we stayed, because sometimes they were lovely and the reward felt good and we hoped that it would last but then the punishment would come and we didn't really understand why.

Transactional Analysis

Transactional Analysis is a simple system for understanding what happens within us and between us. Driver Behaviours really helped me understand why I stayed so long and tried so hard to make it work. The Driver Behaviours are: Be strong, Please Others, Be Perfect, Try Hard and Hurry Up. We were all trying way too hard to be perfect and please him and be strong all at the same time.

Stroke theory explains how we are used to getting and giving attention. It explains why people who have parents who are harsh and critical go for partners who do the same, because it is what they are used to.

The Drama Triangle is the best model ever for understanding the nature of conflict and the head fuck of abuse. One minute you feel like the victim and then the next he's telling you that you've victimised him, so then you try to put it right by rescuing and trying to make it all better but then you end up feeling like the victim again. This model explains all conflict ever.

WINNICOTT

Winnicott is was a psychoanalyst who reassured parents that they only have to be 'good enough' and not perfect. This knowledge helped alleviate some of the shame.

WOMEN'S AID AND REFUGE

These organisations are at the forefront of helping people escape from domestic abuse and their support is free and confidential. They carry out research and lobby for change. Thank goodness for these organisations and others like them.

WWW.REFUGE.ORG.UK

WWW.WOMENSAID.ORG.UK

Women don't have to go through this alone; I urge anyone who feels they have found similarities in these stories to reach out, talk, ask, get help. It is help out there. You deserve better. You can do this.

Julie

Thank You

Thank you to the women and organisations who helped me recover from my relationship: MFCC, Frances Ford, The Freedom Programme as well as my tight, loving and loyal friends and family.

Thank you to the women who were courageous enough to tell me their tales and let me change and use them as the basis for the stories in this book.

Thank you Anita Wyatt for your amazing illustrations and for introducing me to a friend who introduced me to her friend who turned out to be my skilful, direct and passionate editor Kate Taylor. Thank you both for believing in the project and giving of your and skills so freely.

Thank you Michael Piper, Becky Ford and Janet Handley for proof-reading – I hate that bit.

Thank you to Booka Bookshop Oswestry for hosting the launch.

Thanks Sebastian Parfitt for your stunning cover photo, to Su Richards for your typesetting and graphic design, to Andy at Think Digital for your printing skills and Alex Wade of ReviewedandCleared.com for his legal advice.

Seb gave me his photo for free, Mike, Becky and Janet proof read without charge and Booka, Alex, Su and Andy have reduced their costs and gone over and above in terms of their services to support this project. I just couldn't have done this without your generosity and help. Thank you.

Thank you to my soul sisters (you know who you are) who have believed in my dreams, challenged my nonsense, celebrated the highs and commiserated the lows.

Thank you to Gladstone Library and Othona West Dorset for being such havens of peace and purpose for writing, thinking, connecting and yoga.

To my sons M and B, you are my sunshines, and I love you up to the moon and back.

Xx

Julie Leoni, Author

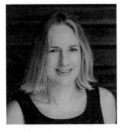

Julie Leoni is a writer, teacher and life coach with a PhD in emotional intelligence, a lifetime of experience in a variety of therapies and a hunger to make the world a better place. She can often be found by the side of a football pitch in the rain trying not to embarrass her sons with her poor understanding of the off-side rule.

www.julieleoni.com

Anita Wyatt, Illustrator

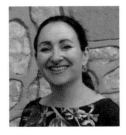

Anita Wyatt in her BC life (Before Children) studied art at Birmingham City University, before working in London as an Assistant Actors Agent, looking after leading actors and attending premieres. She then returned home to her native Shropshire to raise her children and retrain as an art teacher, whilst taking on commissions and exhibiting in places such as the National Trust. In her non-existent spare time, she enjoys learning Italian, running 5kms and driving her children to athletic events.

Kate Taylor, Managing Editor

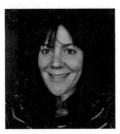

Kate Taylor has been a writer and editor for twenty years, working in the world of publishing in London, New York and Rome. She is now based in Shropshire, where she lives with her husband and two children, running Middle Farm Press. www.middlefarmpress.com